Here are some of the w
Juicing has changed people's lives:

"I lost 15lbs the first time I did the detox with Dr. Etti and 5lbs the second time. I have kept this weight off. I have lost two pant sizes! My stomach is flatter, my face and neck are thinner. Frankly, it is a boost for losing weight for anyone. Etti's technique is realistic and *easy* to maintain."

- S. Cohen

"I have more energy and have noticed a lot of the physical things that bothered me before the program have now disappeared. Aches and pains, digestive problems and fatigue have all been resolved. My wife lost 7lbs and I lost 10 during the detox and we continue to lose weight as we apply the information provided by Etti's program."

- K. Dura

"My body feels much lighter and cleaner; my skin is brighter, softer and more vibrant. My eyes are clear and bright and I have more energy, I sleep better, am more productive and focused. I'm inspired to write and paint more. Thank you so much for this experience, Etti. I cannot remember ever feeling this pure."

-C. Murphy

"When I began Etti's program, I had no idea I was actually embarking on my Journey of life… I have tried other body cleansing programs, but never had the kind of success I had with Dr. Etti's program. I learned so much about my inner soul – what makes me tick and what literally makes me sick. An amazing lightness of energy and glow began to transpire inside of me. *SEXi* Juicing has transformed me and my life! Just DO IT! You will never feel better!"

- Sonia F.

"Going through the horrible effects of what cancer treatment does to my body, I can without a doubt say that without Dr. Etti's guidance and care, it would have all been so much worse. After completing Etti's juicing program, I kept my weight on, my skin never looked better and I slept like a baby."

- B. Long

"Sexi Juicing has helped me get back on a new path of well-being and vitality. I crave healthy, whole and nutritious food that fills my body and soul. It's an amazing process and Dr. Etti is a most amazing person full of love and support for me and her detox groups."

- M. Comer

"Dear Dr. Etti: 'Thank you doesn't begin to express the gift of life and health you have helped me discover. Six days into my juice cleansing and my eyes are bright, my skin has a shine, my hair is soft and although I cannot see it, I am certain my colon has healed. I have energy, happiness and songs in my heart. You have been that Guide for me."

- P. Reizenstein, P.A.

"I have lost 23lbs and I'm feeling great. I'm training for my climb in January and I can't wait to do another detox again!"

-A. Miniachi

"I never thought I could go without processed sugar for longer than a day. But after going through Dr. Etti's WEEK LONG juice cleansing – I realized I could be happier and even have more energy and I know I can do anything I am ready for."

-L. Martinez

"Sure I lost weight, but the main benefit of the program for me really is ONE YEAR of no coffee, artificial sweetener or soda!! I'm celebrating ONE YEAR without all that stuff this month!"

- S. Buckley

"Dear Dr. Etti: I am different today. Somehow your words became my reality. A drink *is* eating. My stomach is the size of my fist and needs no more. Greener is cleaner. I used to be itsey bitsey and now I'm very cherry… While your content was excellent, I think the essence of your magic was your being. The truth be known, I was a meat and potatoes boy who identified with Woody Allen in *Annie Hall* when he's in a California health-food restaurant and says with wry disdain, 'I'll have the alfalfa sprouts.' And I have an allergic reaction to people who talk about eating healthy. Yet you commanded my *trust* by your authenticity, your gentle, playful tone and your style."

-R. Meyer

"Dr. Etti's Sexi Juicing program was a life-affirming and transforming experience on many levels. Not only did I lose weight, sleep without my heart racing, look radiant, I also felt a lightness of being on both a physical and a metaphysical level. The energy I had was off the charts and was never hungry, which amazed me as I love to eat!

I also released a daily coffee addiction that I had for 30 years of drinking four cups on average per day. Prior to this program, I never thought of morning without coffee – and now I don't think of it at all! I feel calmer, more centered and healthier without it.

My physical changes:
- Size loss – Clothes are looser and I went down a size
- Skin – glowing
- Hair – more shine
- Eyes – not only whiter, but the pressure in my eye (I have glaucoma) went down
- Sleep – Heartfelt peaceful at bedtime; before, I could feel my heart racing when I was ready to sleep; that totally disappeared
- Increase in my chi, my life force, which was quite apparent to all
- Broke a caffeine addiction – used to drink four to five cups a day for 30 years

My metaphysical changes:
- I felt far more attuned to the beauty of life and what was happening right in front of me
- Centered in the present moment
- Got more in touch with the "I" in SEXi Juicing
- In touch with my luminousness
- My Love Bucket was much fuller."

-J. Byrne

"Thank you so much for getting me into the (Sexi Juicing) program with Dr. Etti. I felt so much more alive, healthier and stronger. It was a hard yet fun week to see so many people share the same feelings about eating healthier."

-R. Martinez

"Thank you so much for your teaching, enthusiasm and a lot of fun. I AM really enjoying this profound spiritual journey."

-B. Saez

"I am a new woman after SEXi Juicing, both inside and out… breathing deeply and feeling so alive… I am SO grateful for all that you contribute to making your community a very much healthier and therefore better place."

- C. Farnsworth

"I just got back from Disney. Oh my! What a 360 from the vibe of the juice cleansing we just completed! But we managed to eat healthy and I even got some warrior moves in! I cannot thank you enough for doing what you do. The morning sessions and the coming-off-fast breakfast really got to me. I have been flirting with this kind of eating and the connections for years – and I felt like I heard everything you were saying in a different way this time. Your energy and way of teaching and the spirit is so *inspiring* and I am truly grateful."

-S. Gross

"Dear Sexi Juicers:

"Update from the Valme household… We have not had a cup of coffee – in 25 days and we were true espresso/cappuccino addicts. We skin-brush every day, try to do our breathing exercise and certainly appreciate what we eat and how thankful we are about life more than ever. No doubt there are daily challenges, but when we take a few minutes to reflect on what we learned and lean on our inner strength, we are reminded that we can accomplish *ANYTHING*. Oh and of course we try to heart hug as often as possible, which also leads me to share this heart hug story with you.

On the Saturday morning before our final SEXi Juicing meeting and delicious organic meal, I went to our 18 year old daughter, Chanel (who like most 18 year olds can be quite a challenge) and I gave her the biggest, warmest heart hug known to mankind. After a few minutes, she lifted her head, looked at me and said: "Who died?' And I said, 'No one… we have been reborn.' Thank you Etti, for your love and selflessness."

-R. Valme

RESET YOUR BODY, MIND AND SPIRIT

SEXi Juicing

Dr. Etti's Simple guide to SEXi and Juicy living

Dr. Etti

Doctor of Holistic Nutrition

BALBOA.
PRESS
A DIVISION OF HAY HOUSE

Photography by Pamela Jones
Cover and graphic design by José Luis Sosa

Balboa Press books may be ordered through booksellers or by contacting:

Balboa Press
A Division of Hay House
1663 Liberty Drive
Bloomington, IN 47403
www.balboapress.com
1 (877) 407-4847

Because of the dynamic nature of the Internet, any web addresses or links contained in this book may have changed since publication and may no longer be valid. The views expressed in this work are solely those of the author and do not necessarily reflect the views of the publisher, and the publisher hereby disclaims any responsibility for them.

Disclaimer of Health Care Related Services
The techniques and advice described in this book represent the opinions of the author based on her training and experience. Dr. Etti expressly disclaims any responsibility for any liability, loss or risk, personal or otherwise, which is incurred as a result of using any of the techniques, recipes or recommendations suggested herein. If in any doubt, or if requiring medical advice, Dr. Etti encourages you to continue visiting and treating with your healthcare professionals, including, without limitation, your physician.

Disclaimer of Personal Responsibility and Release of Health Care Related Claims
You take full responsibility for your life and well being, and all decisions during and after this book. You assume the risks of the Program, whether or not such risks were created or exacerbated by Dr. Etti who is not a Medical Doctor, rather, a Doctor of Holistic Nutrition. You release Dr. Etti, her heirs, executors, administrators (collective, the Releasees) from any and all liability, damages, causes of action, allegations, suits, sums of money, claims and demands whatsoever, in law, admiralty or equity, which against Dr. Etti and Releasees.

Print information available on the last page.

ISBN: 978-1-4525-9946-5 (sc)
ISBN: 978-1-4525-9948-9 (hc)
ISBN: 978-1-4525-9947-2 (e)

Library of Congress Control Number: 2014921149

Balboa Press rev. date: 10/06/2017

FORWARD

By David Wolfe

I love juicing. Always have. Never felt such surges of well-being until I committed myself to daily juicing. It happened to Dr. Etti, too. At some point she became so charged up on fresh juices, she wrote this book so that she could reach you with the magic of juicing and help you tap this transformative power. Dr. Etti's Sexi Juicing is an inspirational light to help you get activated to take personal responsibility for your health now.

Dr. Etti is a living example of the transformative power of fresh juices. As you read her story I know you will be touched. Reading this book will help you develop the same inner resolve Dr. Etti has developed for her life: to feel extraordinary all the time! That is your birthright. And you can do it.

Fresh, raw juices are simple, natural, loaded with nutrients, bubbling with living enzymes, able to immediately deliver energy and are literally sparkling with delight. If you choose organic foods to juice (and eat), as Dr. Etti recommends, you will not only benefit yourself, you will also help improve the environment.

'You are what you eat' is going to be around for a while. As long as we can bank on that, then we can bet our bottom dollar that drinking more juices is going to make us juicier…and sexier too. Yet, there are other benefits to Sexi Juicing, including:

- Feeling lighter and more limber; in essence…younger
- Spontaneous feelings of happiness

- Energy without calories or stimulants
- More fun with food and more control over food
- Better sex and healthier relationships
- Improved self-esteem and courage
- Detoxification (we are carrying too many toxins; it is exhilarating to let them go)
- Opening up to more strategies for becoming healthy (getting some momentum going!)

You can be thin again. Thin is in. Juicing is in too. And, for that matter, so is blending.

Drinking your food is a great way to manage the fast-paced lifestyles we all seem to be leading. In these pages, Dr. Etti shows us how! Join her (and me!) in the unconditional happiness of feeling The Best Ever all the time!

There is nothing quite like fresh juice. Juicing can get you pretty close to Heaven's gates. Drink the "Love." Get ready for lift off. Now is the best time ever to take action!

Have The Best Day Ever!

David "Avocado" Wolfe
www.davidwolfe.com
Author of Eating For Beauty, Superfoods: The Food and Medicine of the Future, Naked Chocolate
Founder of the non-profit Fruit Tree Planting Foundation (www.ftpf.org)

CONTENTS

PART V: TIME TO CLEANSE

PART VI: AFTER THE CLEANSE

APPENDIXES

For

My children: Jordan, Ellie, Gabriella and Zoe

ACKNOWLEDGEMENTS

There are many people to whom I want to express my gratitude. I am very fortunate to have so many angels in my life.

To my mother, Lea, my first teacher and guide for being a strong woman – I Love You.

To my father, Yehuda – Thank you for teaching me to be generous and open to love.

Special thanks to Jean Bryan, my Spirit Writer, who heard my soul's desire, spiritually channeled my essence, to help write and manifest my words in this book. She spun concepts into words for your healthy journey of transformation.

I also want to thank Pamela Jones for bringing out the goddess in me with her beautiful photos. Each picture shows our successful collaboration and as they say, a picture is worth a thousand words.

And to Haiyun – you are the essence behind every word in this book. I love and admire you, my soul sister.

Finally, thank you to my shining stars – Jordan, Ellie, Gabriella and Zoe - for loving me and being my greatest teachers. I am honored to be your mother. I spread this message of inner power in your honor.

I wrote this book so that other men and women like me, who have gone through painful experiences in their lives, can be inspired and become victorious too.

I have done it – so can you!

GLOSSARY

Affirmations are your conscious thoughts and mantras turned into powerful statements that can create your reality when spoken, heard or read.

Autolysis Process is the breakdown of toxins on a cellular level that releases fat while doing the SEXi Juicing cleanse and is the key to your Fountain of Youth

Chakras are seven major energy centers in the body:

1) *Root Chakra* is located at the base of your spine. It represents your foundation and feeling of being grounded to handle survival issues.
2) *Sacral Chakra* is located about two inches south of your navel. It represents your connections with others and new experiences to handle your well-being, pleasure and sexuality.
3) *Solar Plexus Chakra* is located in your upper abdomen area. It represents your ability to be in control of your life defined by your self-confidence and self-worth.
4) *Heart Chakra* is located in the center of your chest. It is your ability to love and deals with emotional issues.
5) *Throat Chakra* is located in your throat. It deals with your capability of communicating your true feelings.
6) *Third Eye Chakra* is located between your eyes. It helps you see the big picture of life by utilizing your intuition and wisdom.
7) *Crown Chakra* is located on the very top of your head. It is your highest Chakra that allows you to connect spiritually.

Doodles are daily writing exercises you do during the SEXi Juicing cleanse.

Ghee is clarified butter used for cooking that originated in ancient India.

Gluten Free or GL are foods that exclude proteins found in certain grains, i.e. wheat, barely and rye.

G-D is the Hebrew way of writing "GOD."

Gremlin is your self sabotage; the leader of the Itsy Bitsy Shitty Committee.

HP is the abbreviation of "Higher Power" which is an influence greater than oneself.

Hineni is a Hebrew word that means you are totally present with all of your being, physically, mentally and spiritually, to do what is needed in the moment.

Itsy Bitsy Shitty Committee is all the chatter, noise or monkey mind in your head.

Junk & Gunk is accumulated waste and toxins in your colon and other organs that compromise the proper functioning of your body and eventually results in premature aging and dis-ease.

Love Bucket is located around your Solar Plexus Chakra and is your sun, which when sparked, can make you absolutely shine.

Lucuma is a highly nutritious sweet fruit from the Andean valleys of Chile, Ecuador and Peru, used as a powdered sugar substitute that has a maple flavor.

Maca is a powder made from a root related to the radish, grown in the mountains of Peru and is known as a superfood for its medicinal properties.

Mylk is the non-dairy version of milk.

Pathogens are viruses, bacterium or theory micro-organisms.

Pistou is a Provençal cold sauce made from basil, garlic and olive oil to flavor beans, vegetables, soups, et cetera.

Positions are daily exercises you perform during Days 1-6 of your SEXi Juicing cleanse, found in Chapters 18-23.

P&P is an abbreviation for "Plan & Prepare" talked about in Chapter 15.

SEXi is a term that redefines sexy. The "i" represents me – as in the trinity of "me, myself and I" – that becomes one in a spiritual way when you own your sensuality.

Tocotrienols is a source of vitamin E in a powder form.

Vitamin Love is added to everything that we do and say to ourselves and others.

"Youthing Process" is a term coined by Dr. Gabriel Cousens that means slowing down, even reversing the aging process.

100% Organic is produce grown without the use of pesticides, fertilizers or GMOs (genetically modified organisms).

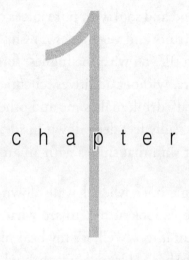

chapter

1

Sizzling SEXi

a t this very moment, your eyes are seductively gliding across these words to see what I am about. Well, ready – set – go. Read it. I am SEXi and healthy from cleansing my body, mind and soul with pure juices made from Mother Earth's garden of fruits and vegetables. Fresh, organic fruits and vegetables that can fill you with the highest form of "energy food" available. It is pure, without additives, chemicals or dyes. So, this pure "energy food" drink makes me and other SEXi Juicers amplify how good we really feel deep down inside, which rises to the outer layers of our skin that shines with an amazing healthy glow.

Sometimes when I walk down a street or into a crowded area, people look at me, to see what is "IT" that I have, because they want it too. Well, it's my health! And thanks to my good health, I have been able to dance through any and all of my life's challenges and situations with confidence and grace.

It was quite a journey to get where I am today. Do not be fooled, it has not been easy for me by any stretch of the imagination to get where I am today. There have been a lot of super highs and dirt-pit lows along the way.

We each have our destiny and we all have the power within to change things around to our own liking. We just have to focus our mind on desired goals because we can succeed beyond our wildest dreams. If you trust and give up your control to G – D, Source, Higher Power and/or the Universe, miraculous things will start to happen in your life.

You are in for a luscious surprise! Faith will lead you to areas in life you never really thought you would be visiting.

Knock – Knock

"Who's there?"

"Me!"

"Me Who?"

"Me wanna be like you!"

Well, well, la-dee-da, Hallelujah! You made it and you are here now with me, reading my SEXi Juicing. So, "Lettuce" be friends and over time, we will happily shed our outer "leaves" or layers until we get to the heart of your life. We're going to seek the pure core of your divine sex appeal – the raw essence of your inner being.

Humans are amazingly powerful creatures that possess a brain able to process information better than any super computer on earth. We also have the ability to discern between choices. Like a fork in the road, we can choose the high road or bump along the low road. Are you ready to shed the past hurts, disappointments or failures plus clean out all the junk that has been taking up space in your mind and body? Do you want to wake-up each day and feel like it's going to be better than yesterday, in fact, it's going to be the best day ever? Well, read on.

In the last fifteen years, I haven't had to deal with weight issues, sleeping difficulties, or loss of sexual desires. On the contrary, when it comes to sex, I feel more sexual and have more libido than ever before. When I do the SEXi Juicing cleanse, I realize that the energy normally spent on digesting uses up to 60% of my body's total energy, which now goes up to my brain and down to my sexual organs. Wow, what a high! I love myself and I love to make love! This is the gift I offer you through this book; the power of LOVE. May you use it to transform your life and to love yourself!

I am going to tell you how you too can enjoy this wonderful feeling of bliss. I mean, a kind of blissful state, an orgasmic kind. If you really want to achieve this blissful state, you can! You'll shudder with excitement once you get rolling on the SEXi Juicy journey. I say rolling, because you're going to have to push through some big changes in order to achieve a true transformation.

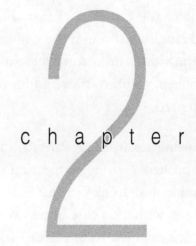

chapter

2

Humble Beginnings

What we are told by people we either love or hold in authority positions, makes a huge impact on our impressionable minds. When you're young, you live in a protected bubble. You just kind of float along doing kid stuff, like playing and laughing through the day until bedtime. Yet, in some parts of the world, unfortunately, children do not get to stay in that bubble of comfort, peace and love, it is instead burst by war, fear or hatred.

Growing up in the rural farming village of Kfar-Saba, Israel, I established a strong connection with Mother Earth. My life was humble and I enjoyed just being outdoors, running around in nature, without a care in the world. I used to love to climb trees to pick oranges. I remember sitting on a tree branch looking up through the branches ahead of me, up to the boundless blue sky wondering what great things were in store for me. I knew from a very early age that my little village of Kfar-Saba was not the extent of my destiny. I always knew, always felt, that I was to outgrow this small, but beautiful place. I knew that I was destined to be of service to others in this vast world I lived in. I didn't know where I would end up, I just knew that it would not be in this village where the orange trees grew.

One of my fondest memories growing up was accompanying my father to the farmers market to purchase our food for the week. I loved going to see all the abundant fruits and vegetables. He taught me how to see and feel the freshness and quality of all the various types of fruits and vegetables. Sometimes, we would be there for hours surveying the goods the farmers had to offer. The colors, the smells, the textures were so vibrant – so alive.

When I was 8 years old, my family moved to Sydney, Australia. There, we also visited the farmers market to shop for our food for the week ahead. I admired the pride of the farmers and the sellers of their goods, how they were connected to each piece of the food. One farmer explained how life energy was connected to the food indicating that it was not only natural, it was also alive. Well, this bit of information eventually transformed my life. My affinity for all things natural deepened. The farmlands stretched out for miles and miles, up and over hills for as far as the eye could see. And the natural foods we ate from those fields were so fresh, delicious and organic because they were free from chemicals or pesticides.

Unfortunately, our time in Australia was short. On the way back to Israel, we took side tours in the Far East. The floating markets in Bangkok, Thailand, where goods were sold from boats were the wildest thing I ever saw. Shopping by boat, I also saw so many exotic fruits and vegetables. Children swam underneath and climbed onto our boat to pose for a picture and beg for money. During this trip, I also saw a little baby crawling on a wooden structure near the floating market. I promised myself that one day in the future, I would adopt an orphan. I fulfilled that promise years later.

Back in Israel, we continued our marketplace visiting tradition. It was a kind of meeting place of peace where the Arabs and Israelis would come together each week. There was much fun in watching people negotiate the best prices, plus hearing all the laughter and shouts of good wishes. Visitors enjoyed the hustle, bustle and the farmers were so proud of their produce.

It was the food from the land that created a true bond of peace among us all. I have such fond memories of taking the time to be with my loved ones and rediscovering the joyful process of making healthy meals that brought us all closer together.

My SEXi Juicing program will help you get back to the simple, joyful experience of choosing your fruits and vegetables, making and feeding yourself with divine living nectars from Mother Earth. It will also help you connect to more than just sustenance for your body, but also energy for your spirit. Food is more than just what we eat, it is the very life force that keeps us alive, vibrant and SEXi.

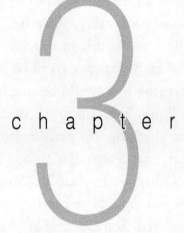

chapter

3

Dance Moves Me

W e all have dreams that only some of us actually get the chance to live out. Sometimes we have to put our dreams aside to just get by in life. That doesn't mean that they can't be pulled out of our memory, dusted off and readjusted to fit into our own reality. Sometimes dreams have a way of unwinding at the perfect time in our life. Dreams and reality can look so different. What appears to be so easy to do for some, is actually something that would be monumental for others to accomplish. Yet, if you have a burning desire, you can truly accomplish just about anything you focus your mind, body and spirit on achieving. Focus and determination are two key components to making things happen in your life. Sometimes it takes a realization that what you thought you really wanted wasn't at all what you needed or enjoyed. Some people are lucky to find alternative roads that lead them to their perfect destination in life. I grew up wanting to be a ballerina. You'll see how that "dream" twirled out into a new life direction. Instead of being the star stage dancing, I wanted to focus my attention on helping others find their calling in life.

Although I was a barefoot "tomboy" that climbed orange trees as a child, I was also very much a little girl. My passion was dancing. At the age of six, I began my love affair with dance, specifically ballet. I remember the excitement I had each day when I made the trek to the ballet school. I had to walk about thirty minutes to the bus stop and wait for the bus. The trip each way was roughly an hour long. While my family didn't always have extra money for lessons, I kept going. Somehow, my parents always managed to find the resources to allow me to continue dancing.

As I worked hard at the dance studio day after day, enjoying all of the sweat and pain, I had no idea that this was another piece of my destiny. Dancing built a foundation in my spirit for my future life in service. It not only fed my soul, but formed a base that I would build on as a Therapist.

One day after dance class, I was walking home from the bus stop in my leotard and shorts. I was 12-years-old and very naïve. My mind was occupied by thinking and talking to myself, when I noticed a man looking at me. He was walking besides me and then seemed to walk away towards a side alley. The next thing I remember he grabbed me from behind, holding me very tightly, with one hand over my mouth dragging me toward the woods. I was numb, frozen. His hand then moved a little away from my mouth, allowing me to scream. It was the loudest scream of my life. The next thing I knew, he threw me on the ground and he was gone. That experience scared me into silence.

I did not tell my parents because I was afraid they would not allow me to continue going to my dance classes. I repressed the incident for many years and I am sure it affected my sexual development later in life. As the years passed, I went through deep emotional work – mainly breath work. I discovered that I had to allow myself to feel worthy and loved and one who belonged. I released all negative emotions from the event and knew it was one of my most profound life lessons.

As fate would have it, puberty hit me hard and my body began to change dramatically. I was no longer a skinny little girl who looked like a ballerina. I began to look like a woman, particularly my butt. It seemed to have grown at an alarming rate. Worse, my ballet teacher told me that I needed to slim down drastically; in fact it would be best that I give up my dream of becoming a ballerina. I wanted nothing else in life other than to dance. I dreamt about the stage and performing, seeing the audience admiring my graceful movements. I was heartbroken and cried for days. It was painful for me, but my teacher would not reconsider. He put an end to my dancing dreams.

I felt lonely and alone. If I could go back to that time, to that young girl sitting on the bathroom floor crying and asking G-D for help, I would tell myself: "Etti, you are loved by G-D all the time, even at this moment. G-D loves you and wants you to know you are beautiful. There is a future waiting for you full of wonderful experiences, happiness and adventure. Lift your head high and know that your heart will attract goodness to you. Open your heart and allow your authentic self to appear. Do not be afraid. Do not worry. One day, you will be loved the way you deserve to be loved; wholly, completely and unconditionally. Whenever you need a hug and there is no one around to give it to you, give yourself a big hug and smile."

I wished I had the foresight to have known then that many of my greatest lessons were the results of my most challenging moments and difficult situations. They empowered me to become the woman I am today. I was able to turn my burdens into blessings and here I am now, ready to help others.

My love of dance was about moving my body to the rhythm of music. In time, I replaced my passion for ballet with dancing for fun and as a form of exercise. Later in life, I realized that dancing instilled a kind of courage and determination to take risks, which resulted in giving me confidence and grace to stand up to my fears, conquer them and move on with my life.

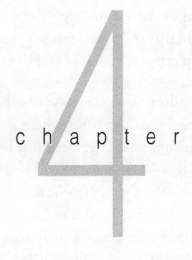

chapter

4

Americanized in the Concrete Jungle

On December 31, 1985, I was a 21-year-old Israeli girl who stepped off a plane at JFK in America. That day, I went from looking up at an orange tree to looking up at the Empire State Building. Wow, what a thrill! I just knew I had arrived at the place I was supposed to be to start my life's work to help others.

As I drove into the massive concrete jungle of New York City, I thought back to being a little girl looking up through the orange branches to see the beautiful bright sky over my small farming village of Kfar-Saba. I knew there was so much more out there and now, here it was, New York City. No matter how much I looked up at the city, I could not see it all. Every time I turned my head, I discovered another wondrous sight. The people, culture and architecture were amazing and magical to me all at once.

Scary? Yes, but in an exhilarating way. I supposed I could relate it to getting on a roller coaster for the first time. I was terrified by all the loops, fast turns up and down, but could hardly wait to get back in line and do it again.

I didn't really think about the date of my arrival back then, but as I am writing this book and recalling my story, it now seems so appropriate that I landed in America on December 31st, the eve of a new year ahead, a new beginning.

I was so fortunate to apply for and be accepted to, the Israeli Mission of Defense in New York. It was a coveted position at the time. It automatically changed my visa status and it enabled me to pursue my education immediately.

I was chosen because I had a very high security clearance from my time spent in the Israeli Defense Forces (IDF). My two years of service in the IDF were rewarding and transformative as well. This was the first time I felt valued and had a purpose. People counted on my performance as an individual. I wanted to be of help, to be useful. I literally worked my butt off and it felt good. I wanted to continue to be of service and make a difference and I knew deep down that it would not happen in my village. Being in New York City was a dream come true for me. In hindsight, I realized that I had manifested this "dream" many years before.

Once in New York, I began looking at colleges. My first choice for a profession was in dance therapy, hoping to channel my passion for dance from my early childhood into helping others. Hunter College had offered a course in dance therapy but just as I applied, the course was canceled.

I didn't know what to do at that point. I remembered something my mother said when I told her I was leaving Israel and moving to America, "You will never make it. You will never get married. You will be all alone and broke." Well, I was alone and broke, but there was no way I wasn't going to make it.

What "IT" was, I wasn't really sure. I wasn't going to be a ballerina and now I wasn't going to be a dance therapist. So, what does a nice Israeli girl do in New York City? Marketing. It seemed to be the perfect creative avenue for me.

I enrolled in the New York Institute of Technology and began to study marketing. Every morning, I would get up very early to start my arduous day ahead. I was on the subway by 6:00 a.m. in order to arrive to work on time. After a full day at work, I would make my way to class for the rest of the evening and then home to study as much as I could before passing out on my little Murphy bed.

My apartment was the size of a large walk-in closet, but it was home for me. It was clean, safe, functional and met my needs. I spent very little time at home anyway as my days were filled with hours at work and school.

As a result of my daily rituals, my diet became increasingly unhealthy. I ate when I could and what I could. I fell into the trap of cheap, low-quality, easily accessible food. My daily meals consisted of Chinese food filled with MSG, coffee and pastries. Each morning I indulged in a delicious chocolate croissant with my coffee.

I continued to smoke, a terrible habit I had picked up during my years in the army. Nothing I put in my body was truly feeding me. My meals were empty calories with no nutritional value. I wasn't concerned with what I was eating, I thought I was really living.

I had little time to socialize. I did have a few boyfriends over the years, but my drive to complete, and pay for my education and survive, consumed the majority of my time. And I missed having family in my life. I yearned for them desperately.

There were times I thought about returning home. Fortunately, I would recover from my "homesickness" rather quickly. I knew that New York City was my new home and that I was meant to be there, no matter the struggles I faced. I would survive! This was my destiny. I was on my path to service. I was not SEXi (See Glossary). My life was not SEXi. I had to hit bottom before I could start to move my life forward. No matter how depressed I got, how lonely I felt, I knew this life was right. I knew it was bigger than me. I could never give it up. I just worked harder.

When I was 14 years old, I had a severe asthma attack that almost killed me. The feeling of suffocation was terrifying. Years later, as a healthy young adult having dealt with that overwhelming near death experience that I survived, I felt I could overcome anything.

We are all very resilient in our early twenties. We can exist on junk food and without sleep or spirituality because we just want to have fun. We can't see our own mortality; it's like a foreign concept to us. We go through life without thinking about our future or our mental, emotional, or spiritual health. I knew I was missing these things. I felt spiritually depleted. I would come to learn later in life that how we feed ourselves greatly affects our spirituality, our emotional health and especially, our physical well-being.

Americanization can be a good thing. In fact, it can be a great thing. America really is the most amazing country on this planet. The American spirit has triumphed over so many difficult times in history. It has been the catalyst for many of the world's greatest innovations. The American spirit allowed me the freedom and access to find my SEXi way, but in the context of lifestyle, it was killing me. I truly yearned to be healthier. I just didn't know how to attain it. If I stopped even for a moment, I might not ever get started again. I lived in a state of sleep deprivation and poor nutrition.

Americanization in this sense has been beautifully brought to light in several recent movies and documentaries. I had become Americanized in the manner portrayed in the documentary *Super-Size Me*. I prized food that was cheap and convenient. On top of that, I existed with no sleep, loads of stress and no spiritual connections. Living in a "concrete jungle," I saw no way to break this cycle.

5

chapter

How Juicy... Man!

a fter many years of my fast paced lifestyle in New York City and just before my wedding in Israel, I felt overweight and bloated. I was looking for a way to lose weight quickly, so I would look breathtakingly beautiful and absolutely gorgeous in my wedding gown.

In my efforts to lose weight for my wedding, I was considering some of the fad diets I had heard and read about. Luckily and by the grace of G-D, while walking down the street one day, I happened upon a crowd of people who were totally engaged by a man talking about juice. He was called the "Juice Man." *Juice? What's so special about juice?* I wondered.

The man had a deep, booming voice and bushy eyebrows. He stood on a small platform. I joined the crowd and listened to what he said about juice, all of which seemed to make a lot of sense. His philosophies really resonated with me. He seemed to know every mineral and vitamin and how each one affected our bodies. His knowledge was impressive and his passion was contagious. It was awe-inspiring and I was captivated by his every word.

Maybe this is it, I thought. *Maybe I can drink this juice and lose the weight.* All I could think about was how good I was going to look in my wedding dress, so I committed to the plan. I drank the juice. The more I drank that juice, the more alive I felt. I strangely felt the little girl in the orange tree coming back into my body with all her energy and vitality. My "juice meals" tasted fresh and nutritious. It was such a healthy, delicious feeling and it became crystal clear to me that this was to be the vehicle I would use to be of service in this world. Unfortunately at the time, I had no idea how to manifest this desire, but I knew it was something to do with health and juice.

At that time, I was working on my Master's Degree in Psychotherapy and on my way to becoming a Marriage and Family Therapist. I had read many books about therapy and counseling and was learning a lot about feelings and communication as well as theories and methods in psychotherapy. I was surprised that with all of my studying and learning, nothing had evoked such a dramatic change in my thoughts and feelings as the gifts the "Juice Man" shared about the benefits of drinking juice. The experience opened up many questions. How did the mere consumption of juice affect me so profoundly? Was it a fluke? Was it magical? Was it only me? Could juice make others feel this way as well? I wanted to understand how the juice worked and why I felt so amazing.

I continued to juice every day. I would go to the market at Union Square and buy large quantities of carrots, kale, spinach and celery. Although back then, I did not possess the knowledge, nor the understanding I have since acquired. I juiced and I felt good, reconnecting to nature, with fresh fruits and vegetables. I was revitalized!

There were only a few juice bars back then. Juicers like Vitamix Blender, Magic Bullet and NUTRiBULLET were not available. The health food movement was not as loud as it is today and the organic movement was in its infancy. The scientific community was finally recognizing that bad food had a direct effect on health and behavior. There were just a few of us "conscious" individuals who knew we felt so much better when we drank freshly squeezed juices.

Not only did I feel great from juicing, I really did lose weight. As I dreamt, I looked amazing in my wedding gown, but juicing had given me so much more. Something had changed within me.

Some fundamental shift had occurred. I couldn't put my finger on it, but I knew I wanted to learn more about juicing. So, I began my quest to better understand how I felt and why I felt this way.

Meeting the "Juice Man" was that one profound "AHA" moment that put me firmly on my path to service. It was my first truly SEXi Juicing experience… and I knew this was something I had to share with everyone.

Juicy Life

Independent of a man's love
Being fed G-D's nectar
Drinking it drop by drop
Feeling a warm caress, soft surrender.

Happy to offer my love to
    You, the Lover.

I give you my heart's yearnings
My passion –
My dance –
My voice –
It speaks your name.

With love, Dr. Etti

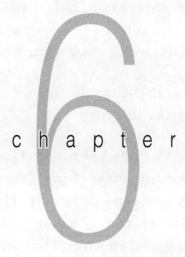

chapter

6

What? SEXi Juicing? Why?

EXi Juicing is about loving yourself from the inside out. Do you love yourself? What kind of answer is swirling around in your mind right now? "I think so – Maybe – Yeah – Sort of – Sometimes – I don't know for sure – Not today – Actually, I haven't given it much thought lately…"

How can you possibly love someone else if you don't love and care for yourself?

As a Marriage and Family Therapist, I kept hearing a recurring theme from most of my clients in relationships – they had lost their own personal identity. They blended all of themselves into their partner and becoming "the couple." They stopped loving and caring for themselves. Their spirits were depleted.

Laws of physics: You can't share what's not there and you can't give what you don't have. Ah… the eternal spring of hope is always available to you – if you seek it. You can always replenish yourself. You can reboot your SEXi self and fill your Love Bucket (See Glossary and Chapter 14). My SEXi Juicing cleanse can ignite your own personal transformation that will reconnect you to yourself again, as well as strip away all the negative connotations you may have regarding the word "sexy." Your cup can and will "runneth" over!

I want to share the definition of Sexy (with a "y"). The definition of sexy means (1) sexually suggestive or stimulating: erotic; (2) generally attractive or interesting: appealing. Since I created the term "SEXi Juicing", I have completely changed the definition of the word "sexy", by replacing the 'y' with an 'i''. The 'i' (or I) is me – as in the trinity of me, myself and I – truly becoming one. It has a more spiritual meaning when you own it. I have guided thousands of beautiful souls through my SEXi Juicing cleanse and witnessed each of them embrace their own individual "SEXi-ness" by becoming aware of its divine essence in their own life... once they understood and owned the term "SEXi."

SEXi is your core essence. It is self-love, a deep, intimate relationship with yourself. When your SEXi has been lost, you must find it. You need to reconnect you to yourself and reintroduce you to your own unconditional love and self-acceptance.

What the mind can conceive – the body can achieve. Even if you don't fully believe in the mantra, you must say it, "*I totally and completely love and accept myself.*" By constantly repeating it to yourself, you will enfold it into your being and in time, it will become part of your essence. As we begin to embrace the concept of self-LOVE, we can begin the journey to love ourselves again.

The SEXi Juicer's mantra is, "*I totally and completely love and accept myself.*" Start saying it over and over again. You'll see, it will change the way you look and feel about yourself.

So, are you ready to embrace yourself and become SEXi? Are you interested in feeling and looking sexier, sleeping more soundly, becoming slimmer, feeling exhilarated to walk through each day with clarity and focus? "SEXi Juicing" is your guidebook to changing your life, complete with:

- Day-to-day instructions through your seven day SEXi Juicing Program

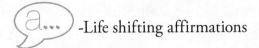 -Life shifting affirmations

- Love Bucket exercises

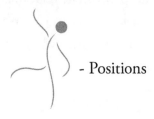 - Positions

- Daily writing exercises or "Doodles"
- Healthy juice recipes
- Healthy tips and nutritional information

SEXi Juicing is a 100% organic juice cleanse, using only the freshest fruits and vegetables, grown naturally, free of chemicals and pesticides. SEXi Juicing creates organic shifts in our mind, body and spirit. You will experience a transformation in the way you think, the way you eat, the way you act and the way you live your life – which ultimately will make you SEXi!

SEXi Juicing begins by giving our bodies and organs a welcome rest and time to replenish themselves. Our skin, the largest organ in the body, becomes radiant, our complexion smoother. We regain that glow we had as children. We begin the "Youthing Process" as one of my teachers, modern day guru, physician and homeopath, Dr. Gabriel Cousens, coined. This occurs when we slow down and even reverse the aging process. Our energy increases and we experience new health, vitality and well-being as we eliminate waste material and toxins from our bodies and regenerate. As Dr.

Cousens explains, "Youthing happens when more new cells are produced than are dying."

A FOUNTAIN OF JUICE = THE FOUNTAIN OF YOUTH.

In June 2014, a study at USC Davis School of Gerontology, led by Dr. Valter Longo, Director of the Longevity Institute, found that the effects of fasting induces the immune system's regeneration, shifting stem cells from a dormant state to a state of self-renewal. "And the good news is that the body got rid of the parts of the system that might be damaged or old, the inefficient parts, during the fasting." Gerontology is the branch of science that deals with the process of aging.

When Dr. Mehment Oz, cardiothoracic surgeon, talks about a subject to better your health, people listen. Juicing is trendy and a more mainstream topic these days. However, I always caution my SEXi Juicers that a juicing cleanse is not going to totally change them in seven days. It's a good starting place, but it must be part of a comprehensive program, a shift in a person's life style. The first step in a conscious change is awareness.

SEXi Juicing is a way of life. While it begins as an organic juice cleanse, it is so much more than just about drinking juice. A juice cleanse is a process that allows the body to relax and go on vacation from digesting solid foods. While on this much needed vacation, your digestion process slows way down, allowing your body to secrete and rid itself of toxins. Juice fasting forces the body to use glucose, fat and ketones that have been stored up over time.

Your body will actually "digest" toxins and shed them through your waste. It's a physiological process call **autolysis;** you lose the weight of waste. It is a purging process of junk and gunk accumulated over many years of eating. Just think about how long it has taken you to accumulate all this junk and gunk... a lifetime! So, when you begin the SEXi Juicing cleanse, be patient, consistent and reasonable with your expectations. I encourage my SEXi Juicers to do a seven day cleansing program more frequently in relationship to their age. For example: Two times a year for people in their late twenties. Three times a year for people in their thirties and four times a year for people in their forties and so on. Once they have achieved optimal health, all age groups only need to cleanse twice a year, for seven days each time.

We take better care of our automobiles than we do our personal health and well-being. I know that most of us change the oil in our cars every three to five thousand miles. What about our bodies, our minds and our souls?

The Dalai Lama, when asked what surprised him the most about humanity, said: "Man. Because he sacrifices his health in order to make money. Then he sacrifices money to recuperate his health. And then, he is so anxious about the future that he does not enjoy the present; the result being that he does not live in the present or the future; he lives as if he is never going to die and then dies having never really lived."

Millions of people are suffering from an epidemic that modern medicine does not know how to cure. They hear the "yelling" (symptoms), but they cannot decode it, or interpret it.

The definition of health in America – is the absence of disease. So, if YOU don't have cancer, diabetes, heart disease or a mental disorder – You are "HEALTHY."

What about all these people who are suffering from:

- Fatigue and inability to focus or concentrate
- Feeling anxious and moody
- Tossing and turning at night and waking up lethargic
- A lost libido
- A variety of aches and pains

They go to the doctor because something is wrong and the doctor runs a battery of tests all of which come back NORMAL. So, the patient is diagnosed as "WELL." I have met with some of these people, who tell me "I know something is wrong, otherwise I would not be feeling like this… I am not feeling well." There is no pill to lessen the pain, no vaccine to immunize against it and no surgery to cut it out. So, what is the root cause of these symptoms?

Have you ever experienced such symptoms? Have you heard that nagging voice? The one that says, "You deserve more!" A voice that says, "It's your birth right to wake-up every morning feeling refreshed and happy." As you put your two feet on the ground, lift your hands up, feel a sense of gratitude in your heart and look forward to starting a new day saying; *"Thank you G-D for giving me another day!"* You have the certainty that whatever comes your way, you will conquer the challenge and make it the best day ever! Find your Mount Olympus (purpose) and be able to climb and conquer it.

A juicing cleanse is a process that enables your body, your mind and your soul to purge and reset. SEXi Juicing is a guide book for a journey into every cell of your body to purge out toxins, emotional baggage or anything that drags you down. It's a journey towards enlightenment that will create shifts in your life each time you do this SEXi Juicing program. These shifts in consciousness change your perception about yourself, your world and ultimately, your life.

As we travel through the birth canal of our mother, we pop out into the world pure and wise. We even know about our past lives and why we have come here again – to elevate our souls and seek enlightenment. We yearn to "re-connect" to the light that is all knowing and infinite. Yet, the second we take our first breath, we forget. Mythology tells us that each baby has an angel. As soon as the baby comes out of his/her mother's womb, the angel touches his/her forehead and the baby forgets most of his/her wisdom and past lives.

As spiritual human beings, we are born into this world to learn. "Learn what?" you might ask. Learn true love and feel absolute freedom. But in order to learn, we need to experience pain, bliss, joy, disappointments, et cetera. In order to learn about life, we need to stay alive, not just exist. BE FULLY ALIVE –TODAY, NOW, IN THIS MOMENT. Are you fully alive? We are conditioned to protect ourselves, to fear, to separate from others and to create layers of defense around us. From the moment of our first breath, we forget our greatness and our divinity, but the desire to acquire it is instilled in our souls. We just have to release our karma, old conditions, low and slow vibrations or anything that pulls our being down because our soul knows our life's mission.

Our body is our soul's temple. We want to get to the light of our soul, the spark that makes us shine from within. Psychiatrist Elisabeth Kubler-Ross says, "People are like stained glass windows. They sparkle and shine when the sun is out, but when the darkness sets in, their true beauty is revealed only if there is a light from within."

You know all there is to know about your life; you just need to remember. Live foods and organic juices bring a higher consciousness into your temple (body) and help you remember your divinity. Soul searching takes conscious awareness. Allow yourself to rediscover your potential and learn how to empower yourself. Do not be afraid to try a juicing cleanse even though you are navigating in unchartered territory. The only thing that is holding you back is yourself with limiting doubts.

To truly detoxify, you need to release more than just the physical junk and gunk. You need to cleanse your spirit as well. You must flush out negative thoughts and emotions that contribute to what you consume in your diet. In this book, you will find daily writing exercises or "Doodles" that will provide you with a simple yet effective process for your emotional and spiritual journey to be recorded.

In order to achieve your maximum physical, emotional, mental and spiritual potential, I recommend you must start drinking fresh, 100% organic juices and stop eating solid foods for a few days. I recommend six days, as it takes several days to slow down and then stop the digestive system. Then you can slowly come off of your pure juice diet to ideally begin a healthier lifestyle.

Hopefully, after you have finished cleansing, you will enjoy an organic shift. You will choose better food because healthy food will taste better. When you mindfully eat better quality food, you tend to eat less, yet have more energy and find that your memory is sharper. A healthier lifestyle incorporates gentle changes that will lead to improved health and well-being.

What happens when you juice? The autolysis process starts as soon as you stop ingesting solid food and your appetite begins to fade slowly as your digestive system shuts down. The energy that is used to digest food is reallocated to purge (takes 3-4 days) then energize your major organs and brain, which can make you feel euphoric.

While juicing, you must remember to hydrate all the time. For best results, take a pinch of Himalayan salt at least twice a day. Drink only quality water such as distilled spring water. Avoid tap water because it probably has been chemically treated and/or may contain other undesirable contaminants like toxic metal, hormones and pesticides or it may become contaminated by chemicals or microbes within pipes (lead, bacteria and/or protozoa). If you do not particularly like drinking water, you can infuse it with lemon, Himalayan salt, cinnamon, ginger, flavored stevia or drink herbal tea. The key is to make sure you drink two quarts of water a day.

Detoxification usually brings with it a deprivation mentality, with messages such as – stop eating the foods that you like – stop chewing – stop drinking coffee – stop eating sugary treats… STOP, STOP, STOP!

My SEXi Juicing program does not advocate deprivation or hardships on any level. It is a process about making small, healthy changes with baby steps. Radical change leads to radical failure. I have found that when my SEXi Juicers make small, positive changes that are attainable, they tend to maintain them over time. Change your mind-set from "no pain, no gain" to "no pain and everything to gain." You want coffee? No problem! Have Cafix or Teeccino. Want tea? Go for it! Have herbal, caffeine-free tea. Want sugar? Have xylitol, stevia, or palm sugar. Want chocolate?

Have some of my Chocopotion Mix (See Appendix D) Want to chew? Have Xponent 100% sugar free xylitol gum. You can have your cake and not only eat but *drink* it too! You will understand what thousands of SEXi Juicers feel when they say, "Today is the best SEXi Juicing day ever!"

All actions begin as thoughts. I've said it before and I will say it again, what the mind can conceive, the body can achieve. We must put positive, up-lifting statements in our minds and repeat them often every day.

A simple technique that I use with my SEXi Juicers is to have them write down what they want to become or achieve. Just by writing and acting as though you have already accomplished your goals helps you visualize your aim. As self-help author Dr. Wayne Dyer says, "contemplate yourself as surrounded by the conditions you want to produce." I also suggest that you put reminders on your cell phone, computer screen or post-it notes, and place them anywhere you can see them regularly and repeat them as often as possible for at least a month. You are basically creating your own mantra to ingrain positive and successful thoughts into your own minds. Repeat affirmations like: "I am a healthy, vibrant being of light" or "I am a beautiful and perfect creation of the Divine."

These words will act as a constant reminder to stay strong and focused on your goals. They will remind you when you forget or when tempted to go astray from your SEXi Juicing program. They will keep you determined to succeed, enforce your decision to concentrate on your goal and encourage you to love yourself enough to NOT give up. Fortunately, there are many healthy alternatives so that no one has to suffer or be deprived of life's pleasures. Hopefully, you will find that life will give you greater pleasure once you have cleansed your body, mind and spirit of toxins. As the life coach Anthony Robbins says "Nothing tastes as good as being healthy feels."

Your SEXi Juicing journey is about you committing to yourself.

> "When you dream, cosmos dreams through you and yearns for it to become reality! The moment you start dreaming, life starts dreaming its dream for you. Only when you don't take responsibility for your dreams, life collapses you! Life expects you to take larger and larger possibilities and take responsibility for your dreams!"
>
> -Paramahamsa Nithyananda

Are you ready to start transforming yourself into a healthier, happier and sexier you for the rest of your life? Are you ready to realize your highest potential and change your life?

"Those who have never tried fasting and are not familiar with the physiology of fasting usually think that fasting will make them weak. The amazing fact about juice fasting, which shocks and pleasantly surprises practically all those who fast for the first time, is that fasting actually makes them stronger and increases their viability." – Dr. Paavo Airola, *How to Keep Slim, Healthy and Young with Juice Fasting.*

SEXi Juicing is your own special love potion.

The Beauty of Juicing

We have all heard the saying "Beauty that comes from within" but what if your insides are full of crap? How could you possibly reflect good health externally if you are full of junk and gunk you've collected over years of drinking and eating? Let's just suppose that all things that passed through your lips over the past year were actually smeared on your skin... like all the fried, cooked and grilled foods, sodas, alcohol, sugar, cigarette smoke, drugs, medicine or coffee. What do you think? For sure you would stink! Can you even imagine the putrid stench of all those things stuck to your skin for a year? Yuck! Try to visualize what your skin would look like if all that was spread over your entire body and stuck there for five, ten, fifteen, twenty or more years. Ahhhh!!! Hello—this is essentially what has been happening INSIDE your body, specifically in your colon. Some people carry up to thirty pounds of fecal matter in their colon! How gross is that thought? In fact, the average American carries up to ten pounds of excess fecal matter. Just stop and think about all the fecal matter that has been building inside of you for multiple years, is deteriorating internally and quite possibly causing health problems or diseases right now.

Some of my SEXi Juicers suffer from constipation because their colons haven't been working properly. Your colon and rectum are part of your intestines, which is a long, hollow tube that runs from your stomach to your anal opening. You have a small intestine and a large intestine which is also called the colon. Your small intestine connects your stomach to your colon and your colon attaches to your rectum and ultimately, your anus. A normal colon is about an inch or two in diameter and approximately five to six feet in length.

Some people's colons are so stretched and out of place that they are almost twice as long and twice as large in diameter as they should be normally. The U.S. National Institute of Health published a survey showing that 4.5 million Americans are constipated most of the time, if not all of the time. In the USA, over 2.5 million doctor visits per year are made by patients who complain of constipation. Due to complications caused by fecal impaction (constipation), 92,000 hospitalizations resulted. Parts of their colon didn't function properly due to a buildup of sludge that stuck to the interior lining of the colon's tube or passage, not allowing fecal matter to move through to the rectum and out of the anus. What goes in, must come out...eventually and the sooner the better! That is one of the reasons naturopaths say, "Death starts in the colon."

Delaying the passing of the toxic fecal matter may lead to numerous health conditions caused by *autointoxication* - self-poisoning by absorbing toxins and clogging the walls of the intestines and colon with hardened waste from rancid foods.

It is said that when the beloved singer/actor Elvis Presley died, the autopsy revealed that his bloated body contained impacted fecal matter in his digestive tract. According to his autopsy, Elvis' colon was five to six inches in diameter and eight to nine feet in length, which is double the size of a normal colon. Stool that had been in his colon for four or five months was also found during his autopsy due to the poor motility of his bowels. He was constipated to the point where he would go weeks without going to the bathroom to relieve his bowels. No amount of laxatives would have helped. Dr. George Nichopoulos, who acted as Elvis' personal physician for the last 12 years of his life, claims chronic constipation killed Elvis in his book, *The King and Dr. Nick*.

In a 2010 Fox News interview, Dr. Nichopoulos stated, "We didn't realize until the autopsy that his constipation was as bad-we knew it was hard for us to treat, but we didn't realize what it had done."

Most people's bodies are full of old layers of fats, starches and proteins in the form of mucus, feces, gases and toxins. Some people have had bacteria, fungi, yeast and parasites that grow by feeding on feces and can excrete their own poisons. Also chemically treated tap water, food preservatives and shallow breathing of polluted air are just a few of the other things that contribute to toxic colons and bodies.

SEXi ENEMA=COLON CLEANSING=TOXIC WASTE REMOVAL

Let's face it – feeling SEXi is a challenge with old fecal matter stuck in your colon, which could cause physical, emotional and spiritual havoc.

I know. It is not a pretty picture imagining yourself lying naked on a bed or bathroom floor with a thin plastic disposable tube stuck in your beautiful bum, feeling warm water flowing in and out of you - plus, seeing all that funky stuff coming out of your body. Yes, I agree, it's not SEXi.

After researching and reading the works of Dr. Bernard Jensen, Ph.D., nutritional expert, Dr. Norman Walker, vegetable juicing pionier and many other doctors, I am convinced that having an enema is probably the best thing you can do for a SEXi, healthy, beautiful body. Giving yourself an enema or having colon hydrotherapy, a colonic or colonic irrigation is certainly worth the healing benefits.

Dr. Richard Anderson, author of *Cleanse and Purify Thyself*, says:

> "These points highlight an important aspect of colon cleansing. Many people, after completing a cleanse, feel energized, uplifted and free of old patterns, thoughts, feelings and memories that have held them back. When a person is on a course of personal growth and wants to change their consciousness but is stuck in old negative patterns of thinking and feeling, there is nothing that will get them unstuck and change them faster than a colon cleanse."

Some energy healing modalities, believe each of the seven major chakras governs a different aspect of human emotion and behavior. The colon's functioning is intimately connected with the base or root chakra, which is also felt to be aligned with the material world, including our basic security, stability, courage, patience and our sense of personal power. When this chakra is under/over functioning or blocked, subtle energy flow becomes imbalanced and dis-eased results. This can manifest as insecurity, violence, greed, anger, constipation, lower back pain, irritable bowel syndrome or a spastic colon.

In my observation, I have found that many SEXi Juicers are more affected by the past than the present. They stubbornly hold on to old negative emotions and traumas, which affect the way they perceive and react to their reality. Usually, repeating the same patterns of negativity over and over again. This behavior is mind boggling, especially knowing that life and our spiritual reality happens in the "Now." So when a person isn't in the "Now," they also miss many opportunities by not being fully present.

Dr. Richard Anderson estimates that, "about 70% of those doing an intensive colon cleanse will recall long-forgotten memories and buried emotions. Often the memories and emotions surface with their original intensity and pass old fecal matter that is purified. As it passes out of your body, so do the attached emotions and in most cases, those particular emotional memories are gone for good."

The next time you consider going to a psychotherapy session, I encourage you to do a colon hydrotherapy or an enema instead. I am not in any way undermining psychotherapy's benefits, as I do believe it is helpful at times. I also strongly believe that some emotions are "stuck" in the body and understanding them will not necessarily bring about healing. Healing starts in the NOW with no past regrets, guilt or shame. Hydrotherapy can be an excellent tool to help you rid yourself of these negative emotions. I know, I am a Family and Marriage Therapist.

Additionally, to achieve an optimal level of spirituality (being in the now - physically, emotionally and spiritually), your body must be pure. Just think about the last time you felt really healthy. Take a moment to remember how your mind, body and spirit felt. You were probably self-confident and eager to face the day because you looked and felt great. You actually loved yourself and wanted to experience life and all its rich variety. You enjoyed your connections with other people in your life, your community and the larger world. Well, I assure you that if you take to heart what I have written and practice the simple ideas and suggestions in this book, you can feel SEXi again. When you cleanse your body regularly and apply my special dose of Vitamin Love (see Glossary), you will believe again that you are capable of achieving anything you put your mind to. This will encourage success in anything you do.

The key to being happy and healthy is you must be clean, inside and out!

Another area of toxic congestion in the body is the lymphatic system, which functions in direct relation to the health of a person's colon. The lymphatic system is the primary waste elimination process in our bodies. When the colon is full of mucus, bad bacteria, undigested foods and toxins, ALL those poisons seep into the lymphatic system. It's our lymphatic system that moves toxins through and out of the body. Dirty lymph nodes are bad news to every organ in the body. Most lymphatic systems become overburdened carrying the garbage from our bodies and cannot eliminate it as fast as needed, causing an overflow of toxins. Thus, the whole body becomes toxic because of this backup.

I teach SEXi Juicers to assess and palpitate their axillary lymph nodes, about twenty or thirty bean size shapes, located in and around the underarm area. Many feel tenderness around these points, indicating that the lymphatic system is stagnate and the body is not able to move toxins fast enough, which causes congestion. Another sign that the lymphatic system is not functioning properly is lymphedema or swelling of the limbs, (arms, hands, legs, or feet), cellulite or obesity.

Most excess weight is poison weight. One of the best ways to get rid of the weight of waste is through a juice cleanse. The only way to drastically improve your health is by drinking raw, organic, green juices to cleanse your body and wash your colon. You will lose weight and regain your health as you discard your body's waste. You are what you eat, digest and assimilate. You cannot absorb nutrients if your colon is clogged. It's like a 30-year-old pipe full of debris that becomes clogged.

Some people call juicing—*juice cleansing* or *juice dieting*—preferring to reserve the word *fasting* for cases of water-only fasting. I use the terms *fasting* and *juice cleansing* interchangeably in this book. Juice cleansing, juice dieting and juice fasting are the same for practical purposes in this book because fresh organic fruit and vegetable juices are used. Very few of us are candidates for extreme water fasting, which requires the supervision of a medical physician. Juicing is a wiser approach for optimizing health.

The health benefits and modalities of juicing have been known for over three thousand years. There's really nothing new about my SEXi juicing cleanse. It's something that has stood the test of time and been repeated successfully. Nonetheless, not all healthcare providers fully understand the benefits of juicing because they may not have recently studied nutrition and/or dieting. It is always prudent to discuss how a juice cleanse will affect your own body, especially if you have particular health issues that require a medical doctor's supervision or care.

Vegetable juices are extremely easy to digest, your body can spend much more of its energy on healing damaged cells instead of digesting big, heavy meals. Drinking only fresh vegetable based juices for a day or two, or even a week, can give your body a much needed rest. This gives your body the opportunity to do what it does best, to heal itself.

The key to your personal fountain of youth and the benefit to a juicing fast is with the autolysis process. As mentioned before, a juice cleanse allows your digestive system to slow down and rid itself of toxins via waste through the physiological process. This happens when your body actually self-digests old, diseased and damaged cells by excreting toxins, some of which are stored in the fat cells. I call this process "losing the weight of waste."

A guided cleanse, such as SEXi Juicing, is a safe and productive way to begin. You will see and feel the positive effects of a properly conducted juice cleanse with:

- More energy
- Healthier skin
- Better quality sleep
- Improved cardiovascular health
- Reduction in or elimination of aches and pains in muscles and joints
- Decrease in or elimination of headaches
- More efficient digestion
- Stabilization to blood pressure
- Normalization of bowel movements
- Loss of excess weight
- Elimination of stored toxins
- Improvement of chronic degenerative health conditions, including autoimmune disorders
- Increased libido

HOW LONG SHOULD A JUICE CLEANSE LAST?

It really depends on your health status and individual goals. If you're looking to give your body a short but beneficial break, it can be helpful to do a juice cleanse for two to three days over a weekend.

If you're looking to experience significant detoxification and achieve some big changes with your health, you might consider doing a longer juice fast, somewhere in the ballpark of one to two weeks. SEXi Juicing achieves the best results with five days of juicing, one day of smoothies and organic vegetarian food on the seventh day, before you begin eating solid foods again.

Although it's optimal to prepare for a juice fast by eating raw fruits and vegetables for at least 72 hours prior to consuming only juices. Most people with good health do just fine starting with cleansing without a pre-fasting routine. For best results, please refer to pre-cleansing instructions in Chapter 17 or visit my website www. dretti.com.

You can drink as much pure, organic green juice as your appetite calls for throughout the day. I have found that most people do well with an average of four 16-18 ounce servings of fresh juice per day.

You can use any of the juice recipes that are listed in Chapters 25-31 or any similar recipes that you create. Just follow your healthy tastes and instincts.

As Hippocrates put it, "Food is thy medicine and medicine is thy food." You are the healer, the lover and the peaceful warrior. You can do it! You *can* heal yourself!

Fasting helps the body cleanse itself of accumulated toxic wastes. During the fast, there is no solid food intake to stimulate the defecation reflex, so natural bowel movements tend to decrease or stop temporarily. Since the colon plays a key role in toxic elimination, it is highly beneficial to help release impurities, wastes and toxins as well as to prevent auto-toxemia or self-poisoning by stimulating the colon with regular enemas, every other day during a SEXi Juicing cleanse is suggested.

An enema requires an enema bag with a rubber hose and rectal nozzle. Fill the bag with *lukewarm* water about 99°F. Add 1 teaspoon of fresh lemon juice. A pint or a quart of water is sufficient for the total volume of the enema. After the large intestine is emptied, some people choose to use up to two quarts per enema.

The more common position for taking an enema is lying on your back on a soft towel with knees bent or feet up on the wall. Hang the enema bag two-and-a-half to three feet above your body to create sufficient water pressure from the bag. To regulate a gradual water flow, squeeze the tube with your fingers.

You may use coconut oil or another organic lubricant on the nozzle to make insertion more comfortable. Before inserting the nozzle into the anus, let water run through for a moment in order to decrease the amount of air in the tube. Then fold the tube in half, clamp it, or squeeze it shut with your fingers. Relax, breathe using slow deep breaths and slide the rectal nozzle past the sphincter muscle that controls the closing of the anus. Continue to breathe and relax.

Take your **time**. Let the water in slowly. This prevents cramping and allows more water in. If you feel discomfort, stop the flow and take a few deep breaths, or massage the abdomen. Then continue the enema again until the bag is empty. If you feel an urge to defecate, expel into the toilet.

If you can, retain the water while relaxing and breathing to overcome the feeling or need to empty the bowels immediately. Gently massage your abdomen. Lie on your back, roll to your left side and then roll onto your right side. Two or three minutes in each position is ideal. If the urge is too much, expel the water and bowel contents into the toilet and try again. Often when the bowel is cleaner, retention of enemas water becomes easier.

When the retention is complete, expel into the toilet. Stay long enough to make sure your bowels are thoroughly emptied. Observe the debris and waste that exits with the enema water.

Important: *Clean equipment* after each use. Wash the rectal nozzle with soap and hot water.

Discontinue enemas after the SEXi Juicing fast so the food bulk can reestablish normal peristalsis (a muscular contraction of the colon).

ENEMA DIRECTIONS

- Add 1 teaspoon of strained fresh, organic lemon juice into a pint or a quart of warm water.
- Hang enema bag at doorknob height and open clamp to test flow; close clamp.
- Dip tip in coconut oil.
- Lie in bathtub on pillow/support.
- Insert tip in your anus; open clip.
- Allow water to flow into colon gradually.
- Massage colon counter-clockwise.
- After a bit of time, turn onto your left side and stay for three minutes; again, massage colon counter-clockwise.
- Add more warm water; turn onto your right side and stay for three minutes; massage colon again counter-clockwise.
- Expel into toilet.

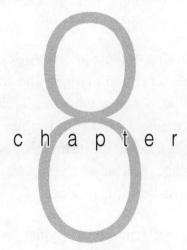

chapter

8

100% Organic Produce
and the SEXi High

t he food we eat contains energy, the water we drink and the air we breathe are full of vibrational energy. So it makes sense to consume as much pure energy – organic energy through organic foods - as possible.

Drinking organic juices provides your body with the purest and easiest nutrition to digest and absorb. When your digestion slows and shuts down, whatever liquid you consume will be absorbed more quickly and directly into your body's cells. So, if you put toxins in while cleansing, they will enter your cells, creating more damage than before. Never cleanse on anything other than 100% certified organic produce.

Organic fruits and veggies radiate sun energy, vitamins and minerals. They also carry wisdom from Mother Earth and from father sky. The powerful forces that come together in liquid food carry a consciousness that penetrates every cell of your body. This consciousness carries the secrets of the ages. These secrets resonate on a high, fast frequency leading to vibrant health.

ORGANIC THOUGHTS VERSUS CONVENTIONAL THINKING

An organic shift in our thoughts especially where wellness is concerned, can bring us back on the path to good health. Conventional thinking is part of what can make us sick. Organic thinking sets the bar higher. Good health is vibrant, it is happiness and it is a deep love for ourselves, our families and communities. What we put in our minds is just as important as what we put into our bodies. Organic thoughts are pure, without toxins and without the ego which blocks us from growing. It is organic thoughts that bring us back to our authentic selves and center us, as well as balance us. Garbage in, garbage out is not only about the food we eat, it is about all of the negativity our minds absorb every day.

If you want to feel depressed, watch the news. I am not suggesting that we detach ourselves from what is happening in the world, to the contrary, we need to stay informed. What about the good news of people helping people, acts of courage and caring? Do we balance the intake of good news with all of the horrific things we are saturated with on a daily basis? Organic thinking is balancing the good and the bad. It is a shift from negative to positive. Positive thinking is powerful and yet underutilized. Powerful thoughts lead to powerful actions. Positive thoughts lead to positive feelings and positive actions. We must choose to feel good every day.

SEXi Juicing and organic living create positive energy. There is a life force and energy force that connects us all. There is energy in every object and atom. Thus, we co-exist with the rhythm of the earth's energetic field. If we consume negative energy, it is inside of us, shaping our health, thoughts and emotions. An organic SEXi Juicing cleanse is one tool we can use to purge the negative energy and fill the space it leaves with positive healthy energy that feeds us physically, emotionally and spiritually.

When you are at your best, when you feel vibrant, happy and alive, you have loads of energy. What you are experiencing is the abundance of positive energy in your body. Look back to a moment when you were truly happy or euphoric. Take yourself to that moment and think about why you felt like this. You were filled with positive energy. You experienced an organic shift within. You can recreate these moments by how you think and string together more moments like these to create your constant reality. SEXi Juicing is an organic shift in your diet *and* your thoughts. Usually the real SEXi "high" comes on the fourth and fifth day of cleansing, which allows your body, soul and spirit to reach a new level of higher consciousness.

When you embark on this journey, you support the culture of life, not the culture of death. You put live enzymes, vitamins and minerals into your body, but even more importantly, you "inject" the consciousness of Mother Earth. This consciousness is pure, divine knowledge that connects you with everything that is alive with the rhythms of nature. You become nature; the tree, the earth, the sky and the sun. You feel the solar power of the sun feeding your organs and this awareness brings you to the right decisions in all aspects of your life. Over the years, my SEXi Juicers' stories put me in awe of this magnificent process of unfolding a new life and rebirthing.

ORGANIC CONSCIOUSNESS AND SPIRITUALITY

G-D saw all that he had made and it was very good. – Genesis 1:31.

When you are with G-D, it is all good. When you depart from your "Source," you succumb to disease, depression and bad decisions. If you are functioning with guilt and shame, you cannot see the truth.

In his groundbreaking book, *Power vs. Force: The Hidden Determinants of Human Behavior,* Dr. David R. Hawkins explains the levels of human consciousness, derived from a muscle-testing technique called **Applied Kinesiology** to document the spiritual realm or energy.

Each level of consciousness coincides with determinable human behaviors and perceptions about life and G-D. The higher your consciousness, the higher your frequency, the more you attract fields beyond your three-dimensional reality. When you resonate on a high and fast frequency, you attract just that, a high and fast quantum reality. That which you think about, that's what you become. When you calibrate at a low frequency, you cannot make constructive decisions. You cannot differentiate between a friend or foe, or right from wrong. **Love** is one of the highest frequencies of being in this world!

Dr. Hawkins claims that the average person cannot shift their frequency much over the course of their lifetime. This idea bothers the rebel in me and it is the reason why I wrote this book. I strongly believe that when you go through the autolysis process, you are able to make huge changes to raise your frequency. When you strip away old memories, vibrations and toxins, you are able to reconnect with the unlimited potential of who you really are. You are able to connect to the "collective unconscious," as the founder of analytical psychology; Carl Jung describes it to be a vessel of truth, love, health and wisdom. I believe that the autolysis process is a gift that is underutilized today because it is used for the physiological aspects of renewal and regeneration. You are connecting to the most powerful Law of the Universe, The Law of Attraction. The most important spiritual aspect of the process is neglected and needs to be further explored. I have witnessed hundreds of SEXi Juicers who allowed themselves to discover their core essence by choosing to fast, immersing in meditation and deep breathing, ultimately going through major transformations.

Individuals who resonate on high and fast frequencies are heart-centered people who have a sense of gratitude, forgive others, praise other people's accomplishments, share and exude joy, continuously seek knowledge and are able to accept change with grace.

Living from a place of ego is constricting and exhausting. Living from beyond the ego, living in spirituality, is expanding and allows us to experience more joy in our lives. Zig Ziglar, a famous motivational teacher says, "You are where you are in your life because of what has gone into your mind. The only way to change where you are is to change what goes into your mind."

- Watch your intentions, as they will become your thoughts.
- Watch your thoughts, as they will become your words.
- Watch your words, as they will become your actions.
- Watch your actions, as they will become your habits.
- Watch your habits, as they will become your character.
- Watch your character, as it will become your destiny.

We can see that thoughts and intentions are the root cause of good and bad life qualities. Therefore, it is important to understand and observe the quality of the thoughts we chose. We must understand the universal laws that govern our lives. This understanding will help us create organic thoughts.

Quiet the monkey mind, the itsy bitsy shitty committee in your head, listen to your organic thoughts and tell yourself:

- Everything I do and say is my choice.
- I am much greater than the sum of my organs, blood and bones. There is an extra dimension to me that is indefinable and infinite. The spirit within me is the spark that leads me to the light – to the truth – and it will set me free.
- I am powerful beyond any measure. I choose to be victorious and not a victim.

- Life is a spiritual experience. I can see my life in the big picture and not get into the melodrama of daily challenges.
- Challenges are here to show me my power.
- Pain is part of life, but suffering is a choice.
- My life is a mirror of my thoughts.
- My mind is a field of unlimited potential.
- Less is more (except LOVE).
- In order to ascend to my highest potential, I need to let go of my negative karma, my baggage. Lifting off in a hot-air balloon requires that I let go of my sand bags.

There is a movie scene in *The Matrix* in which the main character, Neo, is offered a choice between a red pill and a blue pill. The blue pill will allow him to remain in the fabricated reality of the matrix. The red pill will lead to his escape into the "real world."

The choice between the blue and the red pills is symbolic of the choice between the blissful ignorance of illusion (blue pill) or embracing the sometime painful truth of reality (red pill). So, which do you choose? Being brainwashed by consumerism and the more-is-better culture, or embracing the organic consciousness of quality and purity?

chapter

9

You Are "The Secret"

t he film, *The Secret* explains the law that governs our lives and offers the way to create a joyful life – intentionally and effortlessly – by the Law of Attraction.

Simply put, you have to be loved to attract more love. You have to be healthy to attract more health. You have to be abundant to attract more abundance into your life. If you subconsciously believe that you are unworthy, you will not be able to attract worthiness.

You cannot think yourself healthy by sitting on a sofa and wishing for health. You must have a clean slate and erase old vibrations, memories and subconscious patterns of belief. Your mind cannot be unclear. If your mind is foggy and toxic, you cannot produce healthy thoughts. You cannot even imagine yourself being healthy.

In order to let go of the neurotic ego and connect with your spirit, you need to go through the autolysis process, which helps erase cell memories. You have to go down deep into a cellular level to lift yourself up and attract what you truly deserve.

For example, the ego might cause you to think, "I want more, more is better." Instead of, "I am all of creation and all is in me." When you accept the prior statement, you will attract that which is in you.

To work under the Law of Attraction, you need to be proactive in creating your reality and surrendering to your karma and the Laws of the Universe in regard to timing. Intention is holding something in your mind and devoting to it. Under suitable karmic conditions, it tends to manifest. You have no way of knowing when, but you must surrender and allow the results of your intentions to show up in the right time. Any intention you focus on will be manifested either tomorrow or in your next lifetime. David R. Hawkins puts it, "You're responsible for your intention, not the outcome." You must show patience and appreciation. Take yourself out of the matrix, the melodrama, the monkey mind and the mundane daily dialogue to see the whole picture. Imagine you are an eagle. Let the wind take you, trusting that you will fly with grace and land safely.

What do you do if you cannot attract positive thoughts? You might have to do something new initially so you can eventually get to a place that feels good. You might be an alcoholic, for example and feel terribly scared about visiting an AA meeting, but that's what you need to do in order to get better. You may be afraid of being hungry while on a SEXi Juicing cleanse, but that is what you need to do in order to purify yourself so you can use *The Secret* and attract love, health and wealth into your life.

To know the power of the Law of Attraction, you might need to go through some uncomfortable moments, which are based mostly in fear and ego. At these tough moments of darkness, you have to allow yourself to lift your gaze up to the sky and see yourself as the eagle, knowing that you can soar beyond any obstacle or perceived challenge. Look up, "the sky is the limit." Know that fear is only an illusion.

The 13th century Sufi mystic and Persian poet, Rumi, underscores the power of fasting and its connections to intentions and spirituality in his poem:

FASTING

There's hidden sweetness in the stomach's emptiness.
We are lutes, no more, no less. If the soundbox
is stuffed full of anything, no music.
If the brain and belly are burning clean

with fasting, every moment a new song comes out of the fire.
The fog clears and new energy makes you
run up the steps in front of you.

When you fast, good habits gather like friends who want to help.
Fasting is Solomon's ring. Don't give it
to some illusion and lose your power,
but even if you have, if you've lost all will and control,
they come back when you fast, like soldiers appearing
out of the ground, pennants flying above them.
A table descends to your tents, spread with other food,
better than the broth of cabbages.

When your mind is clear through fasting, you work with nature. As a pioneer in America's wellness movement, nutritionist Paul Bragg describes it, "G-D and nature will not perform a miracle until we are willing to bring our lives and our habits into conformity with nature's laws. Fasting cures diseases, dries up bodily humors, puts demons to flight, gets rid of impure thoughts, makes the mind clear, the heart purer and the body sanctified and raises man to the throne of G-D."

Mahatma Gandhi, spiritual and political leader of India said, "Fasting will bring spiritual rebirth... the light of the world will illuminate you when you fast and purify yourself. What the eyes are for the outer world, fasts are for the inner."

All the spiritual masters of the universe share the key to *The Secret* – you can attract what you want to become. If you are seeking the highest and best spirituality, health, wealth, love and joy – the secret is within you. It's in your cells' ability to let go of the past through fasting, cleansing and purification! When you purge your toxins and raise your vibrations, you become the healer, the lover and the peaceful warrior. You become the one that eats from the tree of wisdom and knows how to claim what your spirit desires. You will know yourself and you will own your true divine essence.

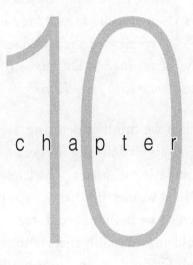

chapter

10

Redefining SEXi

SEXi: REDEFINING SEXY — A NEW WAY OF DETOXIFICATION

"I have made a remarkable observation during many years of supervising fasts. Many men have reported that they have experienced a renewed sexual vigor after seven, ten or more days of fasting." – Dr. Paavo Airola, *How to Keep Slim, Healthy and Young with Juice Fasting.*

When we think of detoxing, we think of health. We don't often think about detoxing for better, longer lasting orgasms and more stimulating intimacy. The latest statistics for America show that 43% of women have some type of sexual dysfunction and 52% of men between the ages of forty to seventy years old have impotence problems. Certainly there is no question that our nutrient-poor and high-fat diets, toxins, over-use of drugs and sexual performance enhancers, plus high-pressured lifestyles lead to low energy and little time for lovemaking. For women, it's becoming an old and all too well known story.

In today's world, most women have to be "Superwoman." It is expected that women must play the varied roles of wife, lover, mother, wage earner, chauffeur, caregiver, teacher, philanthropist and volunteer. The multiple role pressures on women are enormous. Thus, women's lifestyles are energy depleting. Over 80% of women visiting their doctors today put chronic fatigue at the top of the list as their main health problem. Low energy definitely interferes with a woman's love life and sexuality.

A man's libido absolutely depends on the state of his health. A healthy lifestyle has the greatest impact on his sexual ability and enjoyment. Every man can develop his sexual potential to its fullest, no matter what his age. Today's fast paced and highly volatile lifestyle seems to demand that men be "Superman." A man must be strong physically during workouts and sports, supportive emotionally in relationships, balanced under stress, mentally creative and quick, as well as, sexually keen and virile. Whew! It's no wonder that sexual dysfunction is happening to men at every age. It is a real problem. Sperm counts are down dramatically even in younger men.

When you feel sluggish, fatigued, irritated and fat, do you really want to have sex or get intimate with someone? You can hardly stand yourself, much less connect intimately with someone else. Whether you are coupled, single or somewhere in between, you only have one love life and it's time to live it to the fullest.

It is only a myth that people lose their sexual drive in later years. Although we change, men need not experience declining performance, poor responsiveness or lack of libido. A full 80% of men who experience erection difficulty have an underlying physiological problem or medical complication. Most often, erectile dysfunction is a result of poor health or the side effects of medication.

"Bedroom fatigue is not caused by old age, but by neglected, malnourished and atrophied endocrine glands, which are responsible for deteriorating physical and sexual vitality. Premature signs of aging, loss of interest in sex, bulging waistline, all of these are signs of insufficiently functioning endocrine or sex glands and diminished sex hormone production. Fasting has an energizing, invigorating effect on the activity and functions of all organs and glands, including the functions of the endocrine glands. I have heard many reports of the rejuvenating and revitalizing effects of fasting on sexual vigor and ability. Sex urge is motivated by extra, surplus energy. A sick man is a poor lover. All his energy goes on trying to keep going, fighting chronic fatigue and pain. The ill man has no surplus energy left for sex. Fasting restores health, normalizes all body functions, wipes out pain and gives a new vitality and energy surplus. The renewed sexual drive is one of the surest indications that the health and strength have returned." Dr. Paavo Airola, *How to Keep Slim, Healthy and Young with Juice Fasting.*

The power of love is the greatest gift in our lives – it is the supreme expression of endearment from one to another. Love and lovemaking are the most potent expression of passion in human existence. Sexual intimacy with a loving partner brings nurturing and healing energy into our lives. It restores us physically, emotionally and spiritually.

Does aging mean decreased sexuality? No! In fact, it may mean just the opposite, especially for women. Maturity brings experience and relaxation into sexuality. After menopause, most women feel far more spontaneous and much more connected to themselves and to a loving partner.

After my divorce, I experienced a mini "sexual revolution" and allowed myself to let go of the "good wife" picture that I had in my mind. Finally, at forty years young, I started talking about and requesting what I wanted sexually. I felt I had a second chance to express myself sexually and find out how it felt to be fulfilled. I allowed myself to ask for what I wanted. It was challenging in the beginning, as I was not sure of what it was that I was asking for but with a lot of self-LOVE, I found it. As long as you want to connect fully to your Lover within, the Lover that you desire to be, you have to identify ego centered thoughts and behaviors to allow yourself to let them go. I now enjoy a very fulfilling sex life and deep intimacy.

Today, I feel willing to explore love, sex and intimacy to open myself to the lover in me:

**Open to feel the universe
inside of me
Waves of ecstasy moving
through me
sweeping me away farther and farther
deeper into myself
and I find that the ocean is
inside of me.**
- Dr. Etti –

Women suffer today from the "being lost" syndrome. Not really knowing where to turn and losing their core essence of being a Goddess. The divine glorious nectar that is the fluid of life – *Ojas* is a Sanskrit word, which literally means "vigor." According to the principles of Ayurveda, it is the essential energy of the body, which can be equated, with the "fluid of life." It's the birth right of every one to feel SEXi – to connect with the deepest core of who they are and what they are truly hungry for and be able to communicate it to themselves and their intimate partner.

The sad truth is that many people do not realize that the act of making love is much more than just intercourse. Sex is the source of our life force. According to Sigmund Freud, father of psychoanalysis, the sex drive is our most important force – it's the "oomph" that powers our psyches. He called it *libido*, the Latin word for "I desire." SEXi with an "i" also means, "I desire." However, before one can want sex, one must feel SEXi and the quality or act of feeling SEXi is how you perceive yourself and your reality every moment of your life – it's about being holistically SEXi. In other words, being SEXi is the first and foremost relationship you have with yourself. It starts by taking a good look in the mirror finding the lover inside of you and then making love to your divine essence. Love yourself! That is where deep transformation starts, by first going deep down and dirty into your cellular level to clean out the accumulated toxins with the juice cleanse and then reaching that divine place within yourself. It starts by having a loving relationship with yourself. It's all about me, myself and I. The trinity of thy self!

My SEXi Juicers, Danny and Mira (not their real names), have suffered from "bedroom fatigue" for nearly four years. Danny started having lower back problems due to gaining 30 pounds and just did not feel up to having sex with Mira. On the sixth day of their SEXi Juicing, Mira came in to our session smiling from ear to ear, looking radiant and ten years younger. Danny couldn't stop smiling either. He confessed that for the first time in years, he experienced a sex surge and had intercourse that lasted a long time. The next morning his wife Mira told him, "Whatever is in that juice, you should have more of it." Mira asked to me to extend her husband's cleanse for an additional five days.

It reminded me of the scene from the movie, "*When Harry met Sally*," where Sally is faking her orgasm in the restaurant. One of the women who had overheard Sally's "ahhhs and ooohs" said to the waitress, "I'll have what she is having." Well, what you want is the JUICE. That juicy juice that will awaken every fiber of your being and shake you inside so deeply that you are not only able to think about making love, but willing and able, whenever and wherever you wish.

SELF – ACCEPTANCE, HINÉNI AND SEXI – "I AM THAT I AM"

If you want more intimacy, better sex and to reach the Mt. Olympus of orgasmic bliss, you need to examine your relationship with your own body, mind and spirit by asking yourself these questions:

- Who am I?
- How am I?
- How do I perceive myself?
- Do I love and accept myself totally and completely?
- Am I taking good care of myself?
- Am I being gentle, caring and loving to myself?

Then you must remind yourself of the following mantras:

- I am worthy
- I am loved
- I am safe
- I am enough
- I am blessed
- I am divine
- I am beautiful
- I am_____

Tell yourself, "I am here – *hinéni*. I am here with all of my being. I am present with my body, heart, mind and soul, to fulfill my unlimited potential, to serve, to love and to be loved." These words suggest something more than mere physical presence. The Hebrew word *hinéni* means, "I am here with all of my being, physically and spiritually, ready to do what I need to do and to be fully present in the moment."

Many of us have had the experience of having a meal with someone who answers their cell phone, sends a text, or maybe even sends out a tweet in the middle of a conversation. They may be with us physically, but they are not completely with us as their minds have transported them somewhere else. They're not *hinéni*, not present.

"I am that I am" is the English translation of the Hebrew phrase, "*Ehyeh asher ehyeh*," which literally translates as "I will be what I will be. I am the beginning, I am the ending, I am infinite. I am pure consciousness. I am the universe. I am everything. Everything is mine. I am the body. The body is mine. I am the soul and the spirit. The soul and the spirit are mine. I am the creator of all things and all things are mine. I am the window of the soul. The soul is me."

Dr. David Hawkins, philosopher says: "The true destiny of man is to realize the truth of the divinity of one's source and creator which is ever present within that, which has been created and is the creator of the Self.... At some point, the illusion breaks down and the opening for the start of the spiritual quest commences. The quest turns from without to within and the search for answers begins... We change the world not by what we say or do, but as a consequence of what we have become."

You need to realize that everything you see – the entire world – is simply a reflection of your essence and how you perceive yourself. You create your own reality and the universe is your mirror. You control your thoughts. You can self correct and direct your thoughts. You create your thoughts and choose your feelings, actions and creations. You must choose to connect with all that is good.

In order to see a beautiful image in the mirror you need to create and appreciate the beauty within. Consequently, when you experience total and complete self-love and acceptance, you will be SEXi. The journey for you to discover your SEXi self is what the SEXi Juicing program is all about.

Once you discover your SEXi self, everything you do becomes an act of intimacy. It will lead you into orgasmic moments with yourself, your loved ones, your community and the world.

Love nectar is the food of SEXi Juicers. Your inner juice and the organic juices you drink come together in a divine dance to ignite your spark and carry you into an organic-orgasmic experience.

Get ready for this ride, SEXi Juicer! This SEXi Juicing program will allow you to transform your new mindfulness into actions that reverberate throughout every aspect of your life.

Repeat the following affirmation:

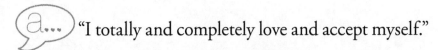 "I totally and completely love and accept myself."

Say it again and again. Repeat it 50 times today and tomorrow and every day from now on.

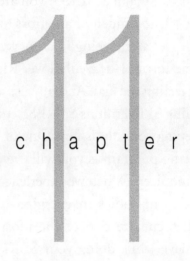

chapter

11

Sleep + Slim − Stress = SEXi

SLEEP

an you feel SEXi if you are tired? Absolutely not, because it is too much of an effort to even think about being sensual, let alone being in a spicy, seductive mood to actually make some form of heavenly love. Right? Well… I have a few secrets for feeling sensual. Actually, it's a formula; refreshing SLEEP plus feeling SLIM minus STRESS equals SEXi! Being well rested from sleeping soundly is key. One of the biggest benefits of my SEXi Juicing program is you will eventually experience a deeper, more sound sleep. When we experience quality sleep we feel better on all levels, our bodies are energized and our minds are clearer. Clarity and focus are two of the most valuable benefits that you can achieve while doing your SEXi Juicing cleanse. Clarity benefits us in every phase of life. Stress takes such a toll on the mind, body and spirit daily. Clarity assists to relieve stress and rid you of confusion in your life. Since the brain is our sexiest organ, we need to nurture it with pure, organic juice "fuel" and allow it to re-energize with revitalizing sleep in order to think and feel really SEXi.

Many Americans suffer from poor quality sleep. This is not only detrimental to our health, but can easily be replaced with more recuperative rest. When you experience restorative sleep, your body takes advantage of its excess energy and actually heals itself. When we are sick, every doctor will prescribe rest. Why do we have to get sick in order to force ourselves to rest? The best time to recover from illness is while you sleep. Conversely, if you do not get enough sleep, you accumulate toxins and can develop chronic conditions such as high blood pressure, arthritis, diabetes, chronic fatigue syndrome, candida, heart disease, asthma, sinusitis or hay fever. According to Dr. Robert D. Oexman, Director of the Sleep to Live Institute, "chronic sleep deprivation, which can occur when you get a solid six hours a night (the majority of adults need at least seven), can lower levels of testosterone – the sex drive hormone – in both men and women… Poor sleep not only affects our looks, health and the ability to deal with everyday stressors, it also kills our sex drive."

Okay, now you know some of the risks associated with not getting enough sleep. So, what can you do to make sure you avoid poor sleep habits and don't fall victim to serious health problems? Below, I've assembled a list of tips to help you sleep, to rest more soundly and wake-up revitalized to seize the day.

Tip #1: Keep a Regular Sleep Schedule

Your SEXi Juicing program will get you back in sync with your body's natural sleeping and waking cycle, your circadian rhythm, which is one of the most important strategies for achieving good sleep. When you juice, you will notice that you are in bed earlier and waking up with the sun.

Tip #2: Make Your Bedroom More Sleep Friendly

The quality of your sleep is most important. If you're giving yourself plenty of time for sleep, but you're still having trouble waking up in the morning or staying alert all day, you may need to make some changes to your sleep environment. The quality of your bedroom environment makes a huge difference in how well you sleep:

- Quiet – Keep noise down.
- Dark – Keep your room dark.
- Comfort – Make sure your bed is comfortable.

- Clean – Check your mattress and pillows to make sure they are free of toxins.

The body regenerates and recharges itself during sleep. Therefore, prolonged exposure to toxic chemicals from your mattress, pillows, linens, blankets and/or comforters when your body is in a vulnerable sleep state, should not be taken lightly. All of your bedding must be clean and comfortable to support quality sleep. Make sure your bedding, including your mattress is cleaned frequently, in fact, get a new mattress every six to seven years.

Tip #3: Create a Relaxing Bedtime Routine

A peaceful bedtime routine sends a signal to your brain that it's time to wind down and let go of the day's challenges and worries. If you make a consistent effort and bedtime ritual to relax and unwind before bed, you will sleep more easily and more deeply.

Turn off your television. Many people use the television to fall asleep or relax at the end of the day. Actually, television stimulates the mind, rather than relaxing it. As you are becoming a SEXi Juicer, try to stay away from negative messages of violence and food commercials. To ensure better sleep and sex, remove the television from your bedroom or do not watch it before sleeping. If you must leave it in the bedroom, unplug it and all other electronic devices before going to sleep.

Sleep positions do matter. For better sleep, try the following positions: Start on your back and support your knees with pillows underneath knees. Try not to sleep on your stomach, as it can interfere with breathing.

Tip #4: Make Love

Making love can aid in good, sound sleep. Making love and sharing deep, intimate moments with your partner eases the mind and creates happy thoughts before sleeping. It is the best stress relief you can truly enjoy. If you are fortunate enough to be in a loving relationship and can share intimate pleasures with your partner before bed, you will be happier, healthier and even live a longer life!

Before bed, try some relaxing bedtime rituals:

- Fill-up your Love Bucket (See Glossary and Chapter 14).
- Read the next day SEXi Juicing chapter in Part V and visualize yourself slimmer and healthier.
- Review our "Pre-Sleep Doodle of the Day" (This is a self-help question before you fall asleep).
- Take a warm bath.
- Listen to soft music, consider my compilation called: Dr. Etti's Meditation CD
- Look at beautiful images daily on www.geoffreybarisart.com.

Sleep "Doodle of the Day"

How do you feel when you wake-up each day? Assess yourself on this simple scale of 1 to 5, where 1 is dragging and 5 is energized.

5 – I jump out of bed each morning ready to face the world with a spring in my step and a song in my heart. Nothing can stop me from accomplishing what I want to do.

4 – I wake-up ready to go and have a steady stream of energy until late afternoon, then I start fading shortly after dinner.

3 – I wake-up without an alarm clock. I definitely have to drive to a coffee shop before I start the day. My energy is high until early afternoon, but I'm yawning by 3:00 p.m.

2 – I usually have to set an alarm clock and often have trouble falling asleep. Getting out of bed is difficult and I drag throughout most of the day.

1 – I wake-up grumpy and immediately need a cup of extra strong coffee. I need lots of energy drinks and sugary stimulants to keep me barely functioning throughout the day.

Healthy people rate themselves a solid "3" and yes, a few rare individuals even score an honest "5." How about you? If you're like the majority of Americans, you may find that one of the bottom three categories best describes you. If so, there's no need to despair – not yet! A steady stream of powerful energy can be yours! It all begins with knowing how to find, make and harness it. My SEXi Juicing cleanse will get you on your way!

SLIM

Can you feel SEXi when you are overweight? Perhaps, but you'll feel a lot sexier if you slim down.

One of the wonderful benefits of my SEXi Juicing program is that my juicers lose weight. Did you know that chemicals, toxins and metals in your body can stop weight loss and bring your metabolism to a screeching halt?

Despite all the weight loss diets and clubs, low-fat and low calorie meals, exercise classes, gyms, personal trainers and diet pills out there, the general population is overweight. It's not news that Americans suffer from poorer health than their peers in high-income countries, a pattern that emerged in the 1980s. This is the norm despite the $2.9 trillion that Americans spend on health care each year, far more than any other country spends. People tell me time and time again that they diet and exercise like crazy, but the weight always comes right back. Sound familiar? You will not lose weight permanently until you get rid of the chemicals and metals in your body and stop putting them back in through unhealthy food, water and skin products. They interfere with the function of all the hormones involved in the weight control mechanism.

Toxins are lodged in fatty tissues and brain cells, but when you juice, your body goes into the autolysis process, which reaches the cellular level to break down toxins and release fat. You will finally lose the stubborn pounds and toxic fat that slows down your metabolism. Your complexion will firm up and glow. The whites of your eyes will get whiter and brighter plus your eyes will look bigger. As excess weight starts to melt away, mucus will also leave your body. Ultimately, when you lose the weight of waste, you will look and feel healthier, your outlook will improve and your energy will increase. Healthy body, healthy mind!

We all know that we are what we eat. When you are depleted of essential nutrients, your body will be in a state of constant craving and trying to shed weight will be a losing battle. You have to nourish your body with living foods and superfoods (refer to Appendix C) that will provide you with the optimal level of nutrition to not only sustain you, but also provide you with vigor and stamina to create the best, sexiest life ever!

We, as Americans, have the right and the power to change.

Philadelphia was rated as one of the 10 largest cities to have a high incidence of obesity. The Public Health Department has teamed up with Food Trust, a nonprofit organization, to establish a "Healthy Corner Store Initiative" that stocks corner stores with staples for a healthy diet, such as fruits, vegetables, low-fat dairy and whole grains.

As David Katz, Director of the Yale-Griffin Prevention Research Center likes to say, health hinges on "feet, forks and fingers" (the last of these referring to smoking). He said, "The power over health resides with each of us as individuals, not with health professionals. We keep waiting for the next Nobel Prize to grant us vitality or longer life, while squandering the power we have to give ourselves those same gifts every day."

Fasting is the key to reducing inflammation, stabilizing insulin levels and normalizing the hunger craving, all of which directly contributes to weight loss. You hold the key to a vibrant SEXi juicy life. Just put down the fork and grab a juice, it's that simple.

STRESS

Today's number one killer comes in the form of stress. It affects us all. Stress materializes in all aspects of overall wellness. It causes high blood pressure, diabetes, cancer, heart disease, skin disorders, asthma, vision problems, circulatory maladies, emotional disabilities and mental disorders.

Stress has been clinically related to obesity and insomnia. So to truly become SEXi, we need to manage, minimize and rid ourselves of stress. Cleansing is a great way to begin the reduction of stress within the body. Cleansing ourselves physically, emotionally and spiritually will immediately reduce stress. One of the key elements to SEXi Juicing is learning how to identify your stress factors and then how to manage them and ultimately get rid of these silent killers.

In our fast paced lives full of pressures, we may feel totally stressed out. We all have to live with stress but if not reined in, it can profoundly affect both mind and body. Fortunately, you can gain control of your life, slow things down and curb your stress. Because stress is silent, we accumulate too much of it before the harmful effects reveal themselves and then it is sometimes too late to correct. It does a lot of damage to our body, mind and spirit, plus has an adverse effect on our cellular level.

Stress doesn't just arise from unpleasant, aggravating times. Positive events such as getting married, starting a new job, pregnancy or winning an election can also raise your stress level.

Stress isn't completely negative. In fact, it protects us in many instances by priming the body to react quickly to adverse situations. The primal fight or flight response helped keep humans alive in their demanding environments requiring quick physical reactions in response to threats. We are not being chased through the jungle by wild tigers. Our tigers are our jobs and relationships and our jungles are the hustle and bustle of the cities we live in.

Today, the body's stress response is triggered regularly, even though our lives are not in danger and this constant exposure to stress factors has an effect on our hormones and can damage the body. Everything from headaches, upset stomach, skin rashes, hair loss, racing heartbeat, back pain and muscle aches can be stress related.

The perception of stress is highly individualized. What jangles your friend's nerves may not faze you and vice versa. In other words, what matters most is not what happens to you, but how you react to what happens to you.

Chronic Oxidative Stress

Unlike acute oxidative stress, chronic oxidative stress burdens the body and causes inflammation, excess body fat, metabolic disorders and premature aging. As a by-product of digestion and toxicity, our inner body is bombarded by free radicals, which are unstable atoms or molecules capable of stripping electrons from any other molecules they meet in an effort to achieve stability. Free radicals create even more unstable molecules that attack their neighbors in domino like chain reactions. Our body is built to protect itself from acute oxidative stress and as it turns out, this process actually benefits from fasting.

SEXi Juicing equips you to handle emotional stress and chronic oxidative stress. Drinking infused juices with antioxidants can actually help you eliminate emotional stress in your life.

To be SEXi, you have to balance and employ the SEXi Juicing formula:

Sleep + Slim – Stress = SEXi

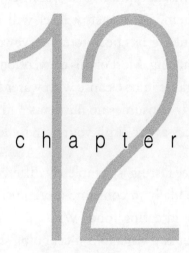

chapter

12

Exercise and Movement

t is amazing how many people believe that, when you cleanse, you should decrease your movement and exercise. It's a total misconception that because you are cleansing, your physical system, your energy level will become depleted. Conventional thinking has been to conserve your energy and take it easy while cleansing. Most of this conventional thinking comes from confusing organic juice cleanse with water fasting. During a water fast, your body consumes no nutrients and eats from your fat reserve, so it is necessary to limit your activity level as much as possible.

Juice fasting is completely different from water fasting. In fact, you are likely to consume more nutrients on a juice cleanse than you would eating food. With all of the nutrition from pure, organic fruit and vegetable juices going straight into your body as fuel, you can actually increase your activity level and exert yourself more than usual. It is only fear that causes people who are juicing to resist strenuous exercise. Your mind causes you to feel tried and sluggish. You simply need to overcome these fears and let your body lead your mind into a new organic way of thinking.

Conventional thinking says "take it easy." Organic thinking says, "Wrong! Get your butt off the couch and MOVE!" A juice cleanse is a great time to move your body, get into shape, sweat out those toxins, stimulate your muscles and fill your mind with new oxygen and fresh, clean blood.

While you cleanse, conquer your fear of exercise and allow your energy to soar! You will have so much more energy than you did before doing the SEXi Juicing program. Fear and bad information are the only things holding you back from moving your body. We can convince ourselves of anything. So, let's think organically and convince ourselves to move.

Bringing my love of dance and reconnecting with my dream to be a dance therapist, I have developed and incorporated my own movements for my private SEXi Juicing classes. They include many different styles of dance; jazz, modern, belly dancing, tribal, Tai Chi and energy movements.

I have been exercising, dancing, doing yoga and speed walking for many years. I remember being resistant to exercise when I first began SEXi Juicing. I devoted most of my free time to quiet time and meditation. Now, after many years of going through the process of detoxification, I turn my ears inward and ask my body for signs. The answers come and I obey. After the third day, I feel like an eagle soaring in the sky and knowing that the sky has no boundaries. I have more energy to run up the stairs, doing it with more ease and grace. You need to tune into your own body's messages. That being said, a juice cleanse is an individualized process. We are each bio-individuals, divine beings; therefore, only you can determine how much exercise and what exercise routine is appropriate for you.

So, turn your ears inward and listen!

To help you hear your body, try putting some music on. Nothing will make you feel more alive than giving your body and spirit over to the beat of music. Go ahead, move and flow with the rhythm.

Research does support the notion that exercising during a juice fast is good for the body. Dr. Joseph Mercola states that acute oxidative stress while exercising is actually good for the body while fasting. If done correctly, you can gain muscle fiber while exercising and turn on the "youthing" genes. He explains, "Fasting also complements the insulin-like growth factor (IGF-1) and mTOR pathways, which plays important roles in the repair and regeneration of tissues for sustaining a youthful body."

Dr. Mercola also describes another study that included more than 200 individuals. The study "found that fasting also triggered a dramatic rise in HGH (Human Growth Hormone) 1,300 percent in women and an astounding 2,000 percent in men!… The only other thing that can compete in terms of dramatically boosting HGH levels is high intensity interval training."

Ori Hofmekler, author of numerous nutrition and weight loss books, explains acute oxidative stress as:

> "… Essential for keeping your muscle machinery tuned. Technically, acute oxidative stress makes your muscle increasingly resilient to oxidative stress; it stimulates glutathione and SOD (superoxide dismutase, the first antioxidant mobilized by your cells for defense) production in your mitochondria along with increased muscular capacity to utilize energy, generate force and resist fatigue. Hence, exercise and fasting help counteract all the main determinants of muscle aging. But, there is something else about exercising and fasting. When combined, they trigger a mechanism that recycles and rejuvenates your brain and muscle tissues."

So, while you might feel like drinking juice is enough during your SEXi Juicing cleanse, you must also remember to incorporate organic thinking and actions. To see the best results in health and happiness, move your body and get some exercise!

13

chapter

Focus – Feel – Flow

Often there are times when I struggle to let go of thoughts, systems of belief and memories – my baggage. I give lip service to the idea that I have to let them go, release them, but if I am honest with myself, I have to own up to the truth of not letting go completely. They just linger on my mind.

This "baggage" can be produced from a variety of situations; from exchanges that happened online or with people I know, or from experiences or miscommunications in relationships. Often I struggle to let go of financial concerns about paying the bills. In all of these circumstances, I observe myself worrying, holding it in and clinging to that which I cannot control. I notice myself listening to my "gremlin," my mind's monkey chatter, which produces thoughts that sound like a broken record going around and around in my head. I become frustrated and angry.

I know it is not easy to confront difficult situations in life and then just let them go, but I promise you, it's doable. I have picked myself up and brushed the dust off my shoulders and created the Focus – Feel – Flow process to help you. It's an approach you can apply anytime and anywhere and you do not need any special equipment to perform it.

As soon as you recognize that your gremlin is starting to do a number on your mind, it can send you into a downward spiral towards depression, anxiety, heart attack and old age quickly. This is the perfect moment to stop and use the Focus – Feel – Flow process.

FOCUS - JUST DO IT!

Stop and observe your thoughts. Take a couple of deep breaths and smile, even if you don't feel like it. Just do it! This simple act prevents cortisol, the stress hormone, from spreading in your brain. Consider your thoughts and say to yourself seven times, *"I totally and completely love and accept myself."* This mantra will center you and calm your thoughts and will help delay a destructive response that would lead you nowhere.

At this point, you have more oxygen flowing into your body and brain, which will help you to clearly focus on the situation at hand. All you need to do next is remember that the past is gone. The past is only stories in your mind, like a book that you can close and detach from. There are no benefits to feeling regret, guilt or shame over the past. It happened and it's gone now.

You need to be in the present moment and realize it's the way you act in this moment that will define the quality of your life now. It's up to you. You are the conductor and it's your symphony. You are either going to play it right or create chaos. Don't worry about the future, it has not happened yet. Worry will cause you to experience a stress reaction.

It's all about now, being in the present. Listen to your breathing and only open your mouth only when your breath is calm, cool and collected. There is no heat of anger in you anymore. Now you can listen with new ears and observe the situation from a different perspective. Self-help advocate, author and lecturer, Dr. Wayne Dyer says, "Change the way you look at things and the things you look at change." Notice what is different in you and how things are rearranging themselves differently. Physicist Albert Einstein said, "You can't solve a problem with the same consciousness that created it."

Release your jaw by opening your mouth, keeping the oxygen flowing to your brain and relax your shoulders. You can change your mind. You can decide not to believe everything you think. You can detach from your belief system and allow yourself to experience a moment without attaching it to past experiences.

Your belief system consists of opinions you decide to take on as facts. It's a matter of your perception. It might be something your mother told you when you were a child: "You are fat'" or "You need to work hard for your money" or "No pain, no gain." You know by now that you have been acting and reacting that way, over and over again and getting undesired results. So, why would you continue acting in the same old way? A characteristic of insanity is continually performing the same action and expecting a different outcome.

It's time to put on different colored glasses. Instead of dark, murky lenses, try some green, yellow, rose or whatever color you like and look at the situation from a different perspective. It helps if you don't take yourself so seriously and if you chose to be in a state of peace rather than judging who or what is right or wrong. Instead of reacting in anger over a challenge, you can choose to see that these challenges are placed in front of you so you can grow. Realize that you are creating your reality by your thoughts and your reactions: Life is 10% of what happens to you and 90% of how you respond to it. You have the power. You are a super force that has come here in a divine form to learn and elevate yourself.

FEEL - JUST FEEL IT!

Life is a wonderful sequence of experiences. Some are pleasurable, some are painful but nonetheless all of these experiences make you feel alive and the more you feel, the more alive you are. People who are numb to pain are numb to pleasure as well. They walk through life just barely existing but that is not enough for you. You have become a SEXi Juicer, you want the whole enchilada.

You allow yourself to be vulnerable. You are courageous. It takes courage to be vulnerable. Allow yourself to open your heart completely. It takes self-love to say to life, "I am ready, bring it on!" The moment you allow yourself to feel, you are free. Free to feel life to its fullest with every bit of salt, raw honey or any other spice you choose to spread on it. It's a SEXi juicy life!

You are entitled to feel angry, sad, afraid, happy, SEXi, blissful and sensual. Feel it all. If you resist your feelings, you resist life. What you resist persists. If you resist feeling pain, you will end up with more pain. Just process the feeling, just feel it but without attachment. Feelings are neither positive nor negative, so break away from feeling guilt or shame. What you are attaching to the feeling is worse than the actual experience of feeling it.

Stop repressing, suppressing and living in denial. Sometimes we like to sweep uncomfortable issues under the rug, thinking that the "out of sight, out of mind" approach works but it doesn't. If you do not deal with your issues, they will pile up like a mountain. Mountains can become volcanoes and volcanoes erupt unexpectedly, leaving behind terrible destruction and chaos. It's time to lift up that rug and start facing yourself and your emotions and admitting "I feel _____." The truth will set you free. Hallelujah to FREEDOM!

You will feel the lightness of being after you start feeling all of that is right here, right now. This feeling will take time to process as some emotions are buried so deep that a big dose of Vitamin Love, is required. The power of love will come to the rescue and some emotions may be accompanied by physical pain or pleasure. When this occurs, you will know that you are alive. You can cry or laugh or scream or cry, laugh and scream all at once. Go for it!

Trust that you are not going to die; you are going to live and be reborn. This trust in rebirth is the best youth-promoting serum you will ever find. When you connect to your inner child and allow your diving essence and unique spark to ignite, you will feel your true radiance shine. It is an authentic beauty that comes from feeling your juice of life flowing within. You will be able to climb any mountain, face any challenge and embrace it all.

FLOW - JUST MOVE ON!

Most aware people are able to practice the Focus – Feel - Flow process. They face stressful situations and turn them into successes without getting stuck in negative emotions. Leaders and athletes thrive on moments like these, when all eyes are on them. They immerse themselves in the moment and block out everything else. They visualize the end result and know they can create their desired reality.

It is not the situation that is causing stress; it is how you perceive the situation. Ask yourself how you act in a challenging situation, "Am I reactive or proactive?"

Just as an athlete trains his body and mind to be in "The Zone", you can train yourself to focus and feel it all. As you do this, you will also train yourself to flow, to move on. When you are able to be present in every moment of your life, you will flow completely from moment to moment.

If you are still attached to past memories, you have lost the present moment and then that moment is lost forever. Once you are attached to an experience, you create an expectation of it, which prevents you from purely experiencing it. You stop yourself from focusing on the present and feeling it all. If your expectation is not met, it will be challenging for you to flow. Let life present itself to you. Put your best foot forward, trust yourself and the universe will bring all you need to experience life to its fullest.

The SEXi Juicer's life-affirming philosophy is:

"I exercise the Focus – Feel – Flow process every moment of my life."

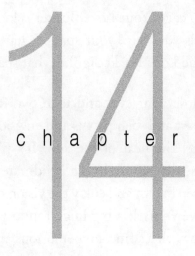

chapter

14

Filling Your Love Bucket

earlier in this book, I mentioned your "Love Bucket." The Love Bucket is the greatest tool in your toolbox. Your solar plexus is located between your navel and the bottom of your rib cage. Your Love Bucket is located around your solar plexus... it is your sun, your spark. That spark is what makes your shine. The Love Bucket ignites that spark.

Close your eyes and take two deep breaths. Go deep into your heart and solar plexus and envision a sun around your solar plexus. Feel the heat of the sun. It's your sun. Feel its radiance. Now visualize yourself as a child. Are you playing in the sand? Take a deep breath and enjoy the vision of yourself as a playful child. Now give yourself a big hug around your solar plexus. If tears start to flow, that's fine, any emotions are welcome.

Open your eyes as you recollect the simple pleasures of being a child.

An important part of filling your Love Bucket is allowing yourself to receive before you give. You know how a flight attendant demonstrates the way oxygen masks work on an airplane? She or he tells you that the first person you need to give oxygen to is yourself, before you give to anybody else, including your children. It's the same in everyday life. You can't give what you don't have. If your Love Bucket is empty, you can't love yourself or anyone else for that matter. When your Love Bucket is depleted, you will feel and look exhausted. You can certainly push yourself for a while but it will further exhaust you and eventually create disease.

The purpose of the Love Bucket is to find what truly fulfills you. Chocolate cake might fulfill but the real pleasures in life are unusually the very simple ones, those that satisfy you and ignite your spark so you can shine in every moment. The shine that comes from within is real, authentic inner beauty. Your Love Bucket should be filled to its brim. It should be overflowing. The good news is that it is easy to fill. When the Love Bucket is full, you feel energized, happy and ready to share your love with the world. You receive in order to share. You never stop the cycle of receiving and giving, giving and receiving. It's a constant flow. The essence of the Love Bucket concept is:

- Live, not just exist.
- Shed the weight of waste.
- Let go of the junk in your life.
- Manifest your dreams.
- Expand your heart and really feel alive.
- Become more youthful.
- Shift the focus from your obsessions to your passions.
- Allow yourself to be all you can be... The sky has no boundaries.

To get you started, here's a list of twenty-five simple ideas you can do to fill your Love Bucket:

1. Look in the mirror and say, "*I totally and completely love and accept myself.*"
2. Give yourself a hug.
3. Smile at yourself.
4. Find one part of your body you love and say aloud, "Thank you for giving me such a beautiful _____."
5. Take five deep breaths. Breathe in love and breathe out any negative thoughts. Do this in the morning and at night before bed.

6. Chose a song for the day, it could be a SEXi song, such as "Sexual Healing" or it could be a happy children's song like "Row, Row, Row Your Boat" (lyrics in Appendix E). Play or sing that song whenever a negative thought or self-criticism surfaces. Then just release that thought into the nothingness from which it came and choose the music of life.

7. Tell yourself throughout the day, "It feels good to be alive!"

8. Appreciate one thing in your surroundings today.

9. Take a quiet walk in a peaceful setting.

10. Imagine it is the day after you have achieved a desired goal.

11. Move to music, shake your booty!

12. Do something creative: paint, draw, photograph, sing, write or play music.

13. Talk to a flower and marvel at its beauty.

14. Do some kind of exercise.

15. Call a friend and say, "I Love Ya!"

16. Think of something you have accomplished that makes you proud.

17. Expect a miracle.

18. Feel the sun caress your face for five minutes.

19. Learn a new joke and share it with someone.

20. Light a candle, make a wish and blow it out.

21. Make a sandcastle.

22. Play with a pet or watch a bird fly.

23. Sit in silence and meditate.

24. Walk barefoot on the beach.

25. Smile at a stranger.

THE BASIC ELEMENTS OF SEXi JUICING

Now you have the background you need to understand some of the processes and benefits of the SEXi Juicing Program. There are many practical, mental and spiritual elements to remember. In summary, here are the basic keys:

- Breathe!
- Drink 100% organic vegetables and fruit juices.
- Drink water, herbal teas and grain coffee substitutes.
- Educate yourselves on healthy nutrition.
- Practice Focus – Feel – Flow.
- Totally love and accept yourself.
- Move, exercise and become active.
- Think and act organically.
- Remember Vitamin L – LOVE!

You are now ready to embark on your SEXi Juicing journey! The following chapters provide practical steps to get you started.

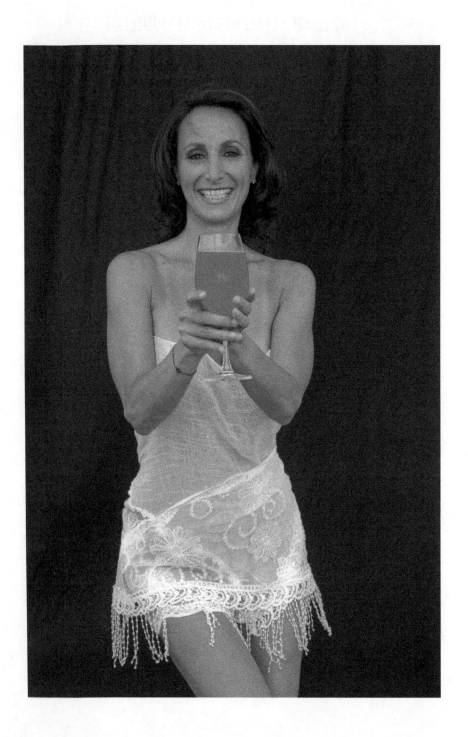

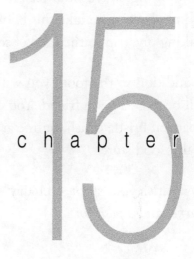

chapter

15

Ready, Set, Let's Go... Shopping

Now that you are ready to be the sexiest you ever, it's time to go shopping! At the end of this chapter, you will find a list of ingredients and recipes for your Sexi Juicing adventure. You might want to take this book with you to the store. I suggest making one trip to the market so you will not be tempted.

In addition to the food, you will also need a body brush, which will become a good friend. You can find the right kind of brush, a natural bristle brush, online at Amazon.com or at your nearest health food store.

To nourish your spirit, each day will feature an *affirmation*, a *Love Bucket* and a *position*.

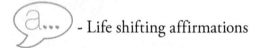 - Life shifting affirmations

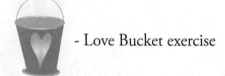 - Love Bucket exercise

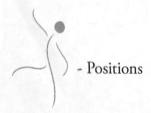 - Positions

Write your affirmation, "*I totally and completely love and accept myself.*" Place it everywhere; on the phone, screen-saver, refrigerator door, mirror or wherever you desire, allowing you to read and repeat throughout the day. This will help you create the new sexier you and help you release toxic thoughts and emotions.

Setting an intention for each day will also free your mind and body to accept the nourishment and experience the cleansing effect has on many levels that will come from the day's activities and juices.

The recipes are simple, delicious and healthy and you will enjoy them four times a day. After one week of this routine, you will look and feel transformed into your most SEXi self. All you have to do is PLAN and PREPARE ("P&P", see Glossary)!

SEXi JUICING SHOPPING LIST

To prepare the variety of juices for your SEXi Juicing program, I have made an overall list with the following "leftover" items for your post-cooked, raw and smoothie recipes that you will prepare immediately following the completion of your SEXi Juicing program. I highly recommend using all organic ingredients whenever possible.

Organic Leafy Greens*
Purchase one bunch or bag of the following Greens:

- Kale
- Spinach
- Swiss chard
- Rainbow chard
- Collard Greens

There are several types of dark leafy greens. It's okay to alternate or substitute greens.

Other Organic Vegetables

- Celery - 3 bunches
- Beet roots - 4
- Carrots - 8 medium sized
- Cucumbers - 10-12 medium sized

Fresh Organic Fruits

- Apples - 8 (Green apples are more tart and red apples are sweeter.)
- Bananas - 4
- Blueberries and/or strawberries - 2 pints fresh, if available. (Make sure they are super fresh as they tend to spoil quickly.)
- Red or Green grapes - 2 pounds
- Lemons and/or limes (at least 12 for the week)
- Watermelon - 1
- Papaya – 1
- Pineapple – 1

Organic Condiments

- Cayenne pepper
- Himalayan salt
- Turmeric powder

Others (All organic)

- Hemp or almond mylk – 2 cartons
- Raw cacao powder or nibs – 1 bag
- Xylitol or stevia – 1 box or liquid bottle
- Raw coconut cream – 1 jar

At eighty revolutions per minute, the low motor speed of the Omega Vert 350 juicer ensures that the enzymes found in even the most sensitive of foods are preserved. It also has a two stage design. The first stage is a crushing of the produce. The second stage is the actual squeezing process. The benefit of this two stage design is the preservation of the natural color and taste of the produce. This also means that the freshness of your juice will last longer. The Omega Vert 350 juicer ensures that you get better juice with less waste. For durability, attractiveness, ease of use, quality and features, it's the best for your money.

BLENDER

A power blender, specifically the Vitamix or the NUTRiBULLET, both make great tasting smoothies. For a list of blenders, see the chart at the end of this chapter.

LARGE THERMOS

In order to drink your juices or smoothies when you are away from home, you'll need a container such as a thermos or large, insulated travel container with a lid. Pre-made juices and smoothies need to be stored in an insulated thermos in order to prevent spoilage. An insulated coffee mug works, as long as it holds the recommended serving of 16 ounces. A 32 ounce insulated travel container is great for two juice servings.

COOLER

If storing of your juices and smoothies is needed for the entire day, the juices/or smoothies can be portioned into four servings poured into four 16 ounce bottles and stored in a cooler. The bottles can then be transferred to the refrigerator once you reach your destination.

LARGE DRINKING GLASS

Get a clear, 16 ounce glass mug to drink the recommended quantity of juice or smoothie. It will save you from running to the refrigerator for refills or measuring each time. Moreover, a pretty glass mug will make your juice-drinking experience more enjoyable.

MASTICATING (OR SINGLE-GEAR) JUICER COMPARISON CHART

Source: Adapted from http://www.harvestessentials.com.

Juicer	Power and RPMs	Price	Juicing Capabilities	Other Functions
Juice Man 408		$110	High speed all-in-one automatic juice extractor and citrus juicer with integrated pulp container	
Jack LeLanne		$150	High speed, large capacity	
Champion 2000+ Household Juicer	540 Watts 1/3 HP 1725 RPMs	$220	Fruits, vegetables	Nut butters, baby food, frozen desserts
Omega 8003 Juicer	246 Watts 1/3 HP 80 RPMs	$230	Fruits, vegetables, wheatgrass, leafy greens	Nut butters, baby food, frozen desserts
Samson 9001 Juicer	1/3 HP 80 RPMs	$230	Fruits, vegetables, wheatgrass, leafy greens	Nut butters, baby food, frozen desserts
SoloStar II Juicer	1/3 HP 80 RPMs	$250	Fruits, vegetables, wheatgrass, leafy greens	Nut butters, baby food, frozen desserts
Omega 8005 Juicer	246 Watts 1/3 HP 80 RPMs	$260	Fruits, vegetables, wheatgrass, leafy greens	Nut butters, baby food, frozen desserts
Samson 9003, 9004, 9005, 9006 Juicers	1/3 HP 80 RPMs	$260	Fruits, vegetables, wheatgrass, leafy greens	Nut butters, baby food, frozen desserts
Omega Vert 350	80 RPMs	$350	Fruits, vegetables, wheatgrass, leafy greens	

BLENDER COMPARISON CHART

Source: www.ultimate-weight-products.com

Brand	Price	Evaluation
Braun Powermax	$60	Excellent at smoothies Good at crushing ice and purees Inexpensive
Oster Counterforms	$80	Excellent at smoothies and crushing ice Good at purees Inexpensive and noisy
Nutribullet	$90	Completely breaks down ingredients in to their most nutritious, most absorptive state
Waring MBB5	$130	Excellent at everything Moderately expensive
Jack LaLanne	$149	High speed, large capacity Not rated by consumer reports
Krups XB720	$150	Excellent at purees and Crushing ice, good at smoothies Moderately expensive
L'Equip228	$170	Excellent at purees and crushing ice Good at smoothies Moderately expensive
Vitamix	$400	High speed, large capacity Excellent at everything Very expensive and noisy
Blendtec	$400	High speed, large capacity Excellent at everything Very expensive and noisy

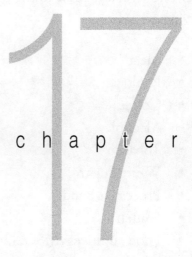

chapter

17

Pre-SEXi Juicing Guidelines

t's helpful if you take time to PLAN and PREPARE (P&P) your body for the seven day SEXi Juicing adventure. Between two to five days prior to the program, you can start to P&P by staying away from:

- Meat
- Poultry
- Coffee
- Alcohol
- Tobacco
- White Sugar
- Processed Food
- Gluten
- Food additives (MSG, high fructose corn syrup, et cetera.)

And increase your consumption of:

- Pure water (8-10 glasses per day)
- Green or herbal tees
- Fresh fruits
- Vegetables
- Natural Sweeteners: Stevia, Xylitol, Truvia or similar
- Vitamin Love

Save your pulp

A special note: While juicing, save your carrot and apple pulp separately to be used in the Apple and Carrot Pulp Muffins recipe, which you will find in the Post SEXi Juicing Cooked Recipes in Chapter 27. You may also use any other pulp as compost.

To ease you into the seven day cleanse program, I have put together a typical pre-cleanse sample menu:

MORNING (UPON RISING)

Slowly sip two 8 ounce glasses of pure warm water; one glass with half a lemon squeezed into it. Do this before you drink or eat anything else the rest of the day.

BREAKFAST

Dice a half cup papaya or fresh fruit salad or make a fruit smoothie. Add 2 teaspoons of hemp seeds. Have a half-cup of gluten free cereal, millet, quinoa, amaranth or buckwheat or any combination, with some hemp or nut mylk. Flavor with stevia and cinnamon.

SNACK

One organic pear or apple

LUNCH

Enjoy one to two medium size bowls of raw or lightly streamed mixed vegetable salad, with a little dressing of fresh chopped herbs, lemon juice, and olive oil. Chew really well to help digestion.

You may add one or more of these protein options: Organic lentils, beans, avocados, sardines, eggs and/or quinoa.

SNACK

One ounce of shelled sunflower or pumpkin seeds or 10 raw almonds, pecans or walnuts.

DINNER

Broil or grill 4 ounces of white fish and steam one and a half cup of brown rice and vegetables. One cup of diced fruit or vegetable soup.

SNACK

Have one banana or one tablespoon of almond butter with celery and/or carrot sticks. Some alternative snacks: Half an avocado with a little lemon or lime juice or raw vegetable sticks with hummus or guacamole dip or a handful of seeds.

BEVERAGE

Drink at least 8 large glasses of room temperature filtered or mineral water or herbal teas such as peppermint, chamomile, Pau d'Arco or other organic blends. It is best to look for bottled water with a natural PH around seven (found on the label) and herbal or fruit teas that do not contain any artificial flavors.

OTHER MEAL OPTIONS

One cup well soaked and thoroughly cooked mung or other beans; half a cup steamed carrots, vegetables or homemade vegetable soup thickened with lentils.

- Do a daily skin massage with sesame, coconut or almond oil after dry skin brushing.
- Do a daily sauna, if possible.
- Do colonic hydro-therapy or enema (One treatment before the SEXi Juicing cleanse).
- Change restaurant dates to movie, theater, spa dates or any other activity not focused on food.
- Unless you are surrounded by supportive friends and family, try to avoid explaining about your SEXi Juicing cleanse program.
- If out at a restaurant or at a friend's home and asked if you would like something to drink or eat, you may reply, "I just ate" or "I'm not hungry at the moment, thank you" and request green or herbal tea.

- Avoid using chemicals on your hair and skin by reading the labels on all your body, dental, personal hygiene and beauty products. Use only organic products on your hair, teeth and skin, including cosmetics during the SEXi Juicing cleanse.

Following is a list of some of the harmful ingredients in personal care, hygiene and beauty products that you should avoid.

AHA (Alpha–Hydroxy Acids)

AHA is often found in the cleansers and moisturizers. AHA is a powerful abrasive that can damage the outer layer of the skin, making the skin more vulnerable to UV rays by up to 50 percent.

COLLAGEN

While your body's natural collagen is good for you, rubbing animal derived collagen onto your skin will not moisturize your skin. It's like rubbing food on your stomach to get nourishment.

FORMALIN (Formaldehyde)

This is the same chemical used to preserve dead bodies. Fumes from formalin have been linked to diseases such as asthma and cancer. It is also a skin irritant and can promote skin allergy sensitivity.

LANOLIN

Lanolin has been found to be a common skin sensitizer causing allergic reaction. Lanolin usually contains pesticides and dioxins.

LACQUER

Lacquer is often found in mascaras to aid in making eyelashes appear longer and thicker; this chemical can eventually result in the thinning or loss of eyelashes.

SLS (Sodium Lauryl Sulfate)

SLS is a common detergent found in everything from toothpastes to makeup. It is so powerful, it is also found in automobile degreasing solutions and commercial floor cleaners. SLS can badly dry out skin and can become a carcinogen when mixed with some other common beauty ingredients.

Affirm to Yourself:

- *Cleansing fills me with joy and energy.*
- *I choose not to eat at this time.*
- *I am successful at fasting.*
- *Juices are super foods in liquid form.*
- *I finally understand how to take care of myself.*

During your pre-cleanse program, I suggest that you take some time to connect with yourself. Calm your mind, relax your nervous system and take stock of all your toxic behaviors, relationships and attitudes.

Try any or all of the following before your start on your SEXi Juicing journey:

- Take a quite walk in a peaceful setting.
- Learn meditation. There is no better way to learn how to calm your mind and open your heart, then to meditate frequently.
- Spend time in a place of beauty, such as the beach, a museum, or a garden. Don't do anything, just observe the beauty around you.

- Try to minimize chit-chat. Experiment with talking only when you have something useful, positive, meaningful or functional to say.
- Write in your journal. Try this exercise of answering the following questions every day of your pre-cleansing program.

☐ What can I do today to truly take care of my body? ☐What can I do today to truly take care of my emotions? ☐What can I do today to truly take care of my spirit? ☐What toxic food/idea/behavior can I do without?

- Do some form of yoga for 30 minutes
- Do breathing exercises for at least 10 minutes a day, especially before bedtime *(See Chapter 19)*.

GETTING READY – CHECKLIST

To make sure you don't forget anything before you start your SEXi Juicing adventure, review this checklist.

TO DO

- Plan menus for the pre-cleanse SEXi Juicing detox program.
- Remove food temptations – making room for healthy options.
- Clear a special space at home to create room for mental and spiritual renewal.
- Rearrange your social schedule. Try to only schedule activities that are not focused on or around food.
  - In case you are attending a social or business function, you may order herbal tea, water with lemon or even a fresh green juice. In order to resist temptation it is highly recommended that you do your best to avoid restaurants or bars for the first three days.

SAMPLE DAY

O	6:00 am	Upon waking lift your arms up and say out loud "This is going to be the best day ever!" Drink a glass of freshly squeezed lemon or lime water (room temperature or warmer). Take one dose of supplements.	See supplement suggestions in Chapter 25
O	6:30 am	Dry brush your whole body.	See instructions in Chapter 18
O	7:00 am	Do 10 to 20 minutes of light exercise yoga, personal trampoline or stretching.	
O	7:30 am	Do enema before showering.	See instruction in Chapter 7
O	8:00 am	Use the provided space under writing exercise or "Doodles" to journal your daily entry.	See Chapter 18
O	8:30 am	Prepare your daily juices (14oz per serving) and recommended beverages.	
O	9:00 am	Drink the first juice (16oz) and pack the rest in three different bottles. Refrigerate the juices	To save time, you can prepare your daily recommended juices ahead of time. Pack the juices in a cooler if taking to work or on a trip.
O	10:30 am	Enjoy a lemonade or Chocopotion	"Same as above"
O	12:00 pm	Drink the second juice	
O	1:00 pm	Do your daily Love Bucket exercise	
O	1:30 pm	Take a walk	
O	3:00 pm	Drink the third juice	You can skip if you don't feel hungry. Always listen to your body.
O	4:00 pm	Enjoy a SEXI Lemonade, Limonade or LOVE Chocopotion	See recipes in Appendix D
O	6:00 pm	Drink the fourth juice	
O	7:00 pm	Do 10 minutes of breathing exercises.	See Chapter 19
O	8:00 pm	Take a bubble bath. Relax and meditate.	I recommend "Dr. Etti's Guided Meditation"
O	9:30 pm	Write your journal entry. Drink a cup of herbal or detox tea.	
O	10:00 pm	Go to sleep.	

ADDITIONAL TIPS

- Adding the cleansing condiments listed below will perk up the taste of your juice and aid your detox process.
- Ideally, you should consume juice as soon as possible from the time you make it. If you must prepare your juice ahead of time, to take to work or for a trip, you may leave the juice in a sealed container in the refrigerator.
- Shake your juice well before you drink the juice.

CLEASING CONDIMENTS

Cayenne	Stimulates circulation, cleanses the digestive system and boosts the immune system.
Ginger	Anti – inflammatory, promotes circulation, boosts the immune systems and aids in digestion.
Himalayan Salt	Helps hydrate and re-mineralize* the body.
Lemon Juice	Antiseptic, antifungal and antimicrobial. Boosts the immune system, breaks down mucus, stimulates the gall bladder and liver. Improves mineral absorption, promotes peristalsis in intestines and alleviates intestinal gas, bloating, pain and flatulence.
Turmeric	Powerful antioxidant, beneficial for the liver and skin. Helps lower LDL cholesterol levels and aids digestion.

*Re-mineralize: introducing trace minerals into the body, which are essential for body functions.

JUICING DRINKING RITUAL

Juices are a very vital form of Prana, or 'life force.' Their life enhancing properties will nourish every cell in your body. Hold the juice close to the solar plexus and take a few moments to breathe deeply before you take your first sip of this liquid nectar.

As you take a sip become aware of how the juice reawakens your body. It gives a burst of energy and a heightened sense of well-being. Swoosh the juice around in your mouth and let your taste buds fully savor its delicious taste and texture. Try to imagine the juice becoming one with your blood and flowing through your system, feeding your internal organs with vital nutrients.

Take your time. Enjoy this unique experience… as the juice jump starts your journey to greater health and vitality.

You will drink your juice in three hour intervals during your SEXi Juicing program:

Morning Juice: 9:00 a.m.
Afternoon Juice: 12:00 p.m.
Snack Juice: 3:00 p.m.
Evening Juice: 6:00 p.m.

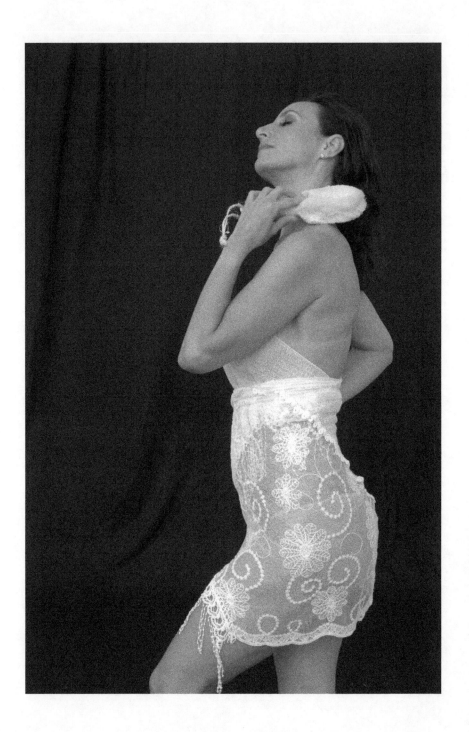

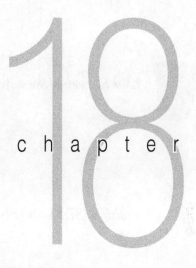

chapter

18

Day 1: Get Naked and Make Love

Affirmation: "I totally and completely love and accept myself!"

 Love Bucket: How will you fill your Love Bucket today?

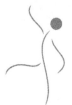 *Position*: SEXi body brushing in front of a mirror.

BODY BRUSH

dry skin brushing promotes circulation and lymphatic drainage, which offers a variety of benefits. Those include: Stimulating the exchange of nutrients and wastes, improving immune function and promoting the flow of vital energy or what the Chinese refer to as life energy, Chi/Qi. It also decreases muscular tension, while improving lung capacity, digestion, bowel movements, blood circulation and lymph drainage. The largest organ in the body, the skin, is stimulated by dry body brushing which ultimately contributes to a clear mind.

Now get naked, stand in front of a mirror and start making love to yourself. First, look deep into your eyes. They are the windows to your soul, to the true you, to your essence. Through the years, your vessel, your physical body, will change, but your eyes and the "you" behind your eyes will always remain the same. Find that person. Know that person and most importantly, love that person.

Every time you step in front of the mirror say to yourself, "*I totally and completely love and accept myself.*"

In order to get in tune with your SEXi juicy self, you need to also be in touch with the outer you and that starts with practicing the art of literally touching yourself with love and care. Dry skin brushing fosters this care by giving you time to make your exterior feel as healthy and beautiful as your interior.

The best time to use your skin brush is first thing in the morning, before taking a shower. Always start by brushing gently and always brush toward your heart (up your arms, starting from your fingers and up your legs, starting from your feet). Visualize your ideal body as you brush and love yourself.

BODY BRUSH DIRECTIONS

Body Part		# of strokes
Fingers	Each side, front and back toward heart	7
	Web in between thumb and forefinger	14
	Palm toward heart	14
Arms	Toward heart	7
Feet	Bottom	7
	Top (like if you were shining shoes)	7
Legs	Up toward heart	7
Neck	Back of neck	
	Up & down scrubbing motion	14
	Side-to-side scrubbing motion	14
	Front toward heart	7
Jaw	Down toward heart	7
Back	Down toward heart	7
Armpit	Circular (first to the left/then to the right)	7
Groin	Round toward heart	7
Sides	Up and down one stroke	28
Stomach	Back and forth (upper and lower)	14
Back	Across	14
Solar plex.	Right/Left	14
Back	Up and down	14
Arm	Around	7
Butt	Circular	14
Kidneys	Back to front	7
Thymus	Double-thump	14

CREATE YOUR VISION

Choosing a dream to manifest into reality is all about bringing your vision to life. You can let your imagination go wild, as long as you are able to visualize that fantasy down to the most specific detail, actually feel being in "The Zone" and becoming totally immersed with your desire. Absolutely anything is possible if you truly believe that focus, faith and action will bring forth what you see in your mind's eye.

You don't know what you really do know, thanks to your innate wisdom or inner eye intuitively guiding you from moment to moment to experience your journey through the roller coaster of living life. Your consciousness is the executive control panel of your mind that invents your experiences and steers your changes. When you tap into your third eye and awaken the pineal gland, it allows your mind to perceive a higher consciousness and can direct your body's thirst, hunger, sexual appetite…and more.

It's like creating your own personal game plan, outlining various plateaus you aim to reach as you scale to the top, to reach your goal. If you're starting at ground zero, you have to map the directions of where you're going to reach your destination. The more descriptive you are with details, the more vivid the day in your life picture will spring into action. Now turn up the energy level of becoming your vision. Write your own unique story with you starring in the lead role. Immerse yourself in the part. Make your words jump off the page into life by you manifesting them into action.

"You must be the change you wish to see in the world."

Mahatma Gandhi

YOUR SCRIPT FOR THE UNIVERSE

Writing Exercise – "Doodles"

Get comfortable in your sacred, quiet space. Close your eyes and take a few long, deep breaths. Turn off the monkey brain and still your mind. Ask yourself, "Show me the best vision of myself." Wait and listen to your heart's response. This a process of unveiling the screen of being "The Star," so if things are foggy…it's ok…just write down what you just saw.

YOUR MENU FOR THE UNIVERSE

Writing Exercise – "Doodles"

Holding onto the best ever image of you, colorfully describe in the present tense the details of every part of your body. Share your true feelings and reveal your spirit. Be artistically passionate with your design of words. You are telling The Universe specifically how you want to look and feel. You may wish to draw a self-portrait or create an expressive collage.

YOUR RECIPE FOR THE UNIVERSE

Writing Exercise – "Doodles"

To manifest the picture of "The Best Me Ever," you have to put some energy into motion. Close your eyes and ask yourself, "Show me how I can achieve the best vision of myself?" While you're breathing, listen to what your heart is telling you. Writing in the present tense, define what actions you must accomplish to attain "The Look" you aim to become.

DAY 4

Breakfast:	Gluten free Granola with Raisins, Seeds and Coconut Mylk
Lunch:	Zesty Corn Cakes with a Mixed Baby Spring Salad
Dinner:	Tomato Miso Soup
Dessert:	Vegan Carrot Cake with Pineapple Sauce

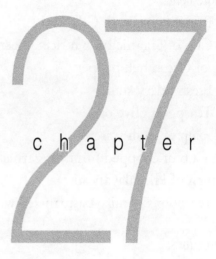

chapter

27

Post – SEXi Juicing _Cooked_ Recipes

BROWN CILANTRO JASMIN RICE

Ingredients:

2 Bunches of Fresh Cilantro
1 Cup of organic brown rice or jasmine rice
½ of Green bell pepper
1 Fresh celery stalk
1 Teaspoon olive oil
¼ Cup of fresh water
½ Cup of chopped mint for garnish
Pinch of Himalayan salt
2 Teaspoons of miso paste mixed with 3 cups water for miso stock.

Directions:

Chop the cilantro and blend in blender or food processor with fresh water. Dice bell pepper and celery. In a large pan, add peppers, celery, cilantro, miso stock, rice and olive oil. Stir, simmer, and covered until rice is cooked. Salt to taste and garnish with mint leaves or alfalfa sprouts.

SIMPLE CARROT SOUP

Ingredients:

2 Tablespoons of ghee or extra virgin coconut oil
1 Onion chopped
1 Tablespoon of red curry paste or to taste
2 Pounds of carrots peeled and chopped into ½ inch chunks
14 Ounce can of full-fat coconut mylk
½ Teaspoon of Himalayan salt or to taste
½ Cup of water or enough to cover all ingredients.
1 Lemon or lime

Directions:

In a large soup pan over medium-high heat add the ghee or coconut oil and onions. Stir until the onions are well-coated and allow to sauté until translucent for a few minutes. Stir in the curry paste and then the carrots. Allow to cook another minute or two and then add the coconut mylk, Himalayan salt and water. Add more water if needed. Allow to simmer until the carrots are tender, 10 - 15 minutes and then puree using a blender or hand blender until the soup is completely silky smooth. This next part is important (with any soup recipe) - make any needed adjustments to taste. Add more water if the consistency needs to be thinned out a bit. After that, taste for salt, adding more if needed. I also like to season this soup with a great big squeeze of lemon or lime juice. Top with something crunchy like toasted almonds or something green like micro greens and cilantro.

BANANA-CAROB CAKE*
GLUTEN FREE

Ingredients:
3 Cups of buckwheat flour or buckwheat pancake flour
1 Cup of flaxseed meal
4 Tablespoons of arrowroot or tapioca starch
2 Teaspoons of baking soda
1 Teaspoon of salt
2 Cups of carob
2 Tablespoons of raw cacao powder
7 to 9 Ripe bananas (smashed)
2/3 Cup of olive oil
2/3 Cup plus 2 tablespoons of maple syrup or 1 cup applesauce
1 Teaspoon of cacao nibs

Directions:

Mix 2 cups flour with flaxseed meal. Add baking soda, salt, arrowroot starch, carob and cacao together. Mash 7 to 9 ripe bananas with a fork. Add olive oil and maple syrup to the dry ingredients and mix. Add mashed bananas. If you prefer a sweeter taste, add 1 cup applesauce. Place in baking mold and top with the cacao nibs. Bake at 350 degrees for about 25 minutes. Slice 2 or 3 bananas into quarter-size pieces. Place the slices on a cookie sheet and cover with 2 tablespoons maple syrup. Bake for 15 minutes until caramelized and let cool. Cool the cake on a rack. Remove from mold and decorate with the banana slices.

APPLE AND CARROT PULP MUFFINS

Pulp Ingredients:
1-½ Pounds of carrot pulp (Fiber leftovers separated by juicer).
½ Pound of apple pulp (Fiber leftover separated by juicer).

Dry Ingredients:
½ Cup of hemp seeds
¼ Cup of coconut flakes
1 Teaspoon of baking soda
1-½ Teaspoons of baking powder
1 Cup of dried blueberries, cranberries, or raisins
½ Teaspoon of orange zest
1-½ Cups of spelt or buckwheat flour
1-½ Cups of coconut or dark rye flour
½ Teaspoon of Himalayan salt
1-¼ Teaspoons of cinnamon

Wet Ingredients:

2 Organic eggs

2 Teaspoon of vanilla extract

1 Cup of extra virgin coconut oil

2 Cups of almond mylk (optional)

1-½ Cups of raw agave

Directions:

Mix the apple pulp and carrot pulps together, then spread evenly onto a baking sheet. Bake at 360 degrees for 15 to 20 minutes* or until dry. Mix all dry ingredients and add the baked pulp mix. Make sure to breakup all the big clumps. In a separate bowl, first mix the wet ingredients and then add in the dry/pulp mixtures. Stir until mixture is like dough. Put medium size muffin baking (parchment) paper cups in a muffing tray. Portion the dough into the muffin cups. Bake at 350 degrees for 15 minutes, then lower to 325 degrees and bake for an additional 10 minutes. Lower once more to 300 degrees and bake for 5 minutes.* Use a toothpick to test if the inside is cooked but still moist.

*Times and temperatures are for a convection oven. Adjust the baking time accordingly if using a regular oven.

SAUTÉED YAM AND VEGETABLES WITH COCONUT SAUCE

Ingredients:

1 Yam

¼ Cup of scallions or yellow onion (optional)

3 Chard leaves or baby bok choy leaves

1 Red or yellow bell pepper

2 Cups of coconut mylk

1 Tablespoon of thyme
1 Tablespoon of basil
1 Tablespoon of rosemary
2 Tablespoons of Thai curry paste (red)

Directions:

Peel and cube the yam and then boil it in water until soft. Dice onions, scallions and yellow peppers. Caramelize onions and peppers in a pan with coconut oil over medium heat. Roughly chop rosemary, basil and thyme, add to the pan. Add the soft yam to the pan, mix in coconut mylk and Thai curry paste and simmer until all are thoroughly heated.

NORI QUINOA ROLL WITH CITRUS CILANTRO SAUCE

It's helpful to have a bamboo sushi mat for this recipe.

Quinoa Roll Ingredients:

1 Nori or seaweed sheet per person
1 Cup of white quinoa, boiled or steamed
1 Tablespoon of rice vinegar
1 Teaspoon of stevia
½ Mango
1 Cucumber
1 Cup of alfalfa sprouts
½ Zucchini
½ Carrot
½ Teaspoon of fresh ginger, minced

Quinoa Roll Directions:

Cook quinoa according to the package directions; do not add salt or olive oil to the water.

Let quinoa cool. Julienne the mangos, zucchini, carrot and cucumber. In a different bowl, mix rice vinegar and stevia. Add this mixture to the quinoa and mix everything with your hands. Before you start to make the sushi, fill a bowl with fresh water and 1/3 cup rice vinegar. Use this water to wet your hands before making each roll. Put a Nori sheet on a dry surface of cutting board or bamboo sushi mat. Take a handful of quinoa and spread it on the first quarter of the Nori sheet. Put 4 pieces of each vegetable and mango on top of the quinoa. Add a little minced ginger and top with alfalfa sprouts. Roll using a bamboo sushi mat.

Citrus Cilantro Sauce Ingredients:

1 Cup of Orange Juice
1 Tablespoon of Lemon Juice
1 Bunch of fresh cilantro
1 Teaspoon of orange zest
1 Teaspoon of honey
Olive oil and sesame oil to taste
Salt and pepper to taste.

Directions:

Mix vinegar, honey and citrus juices, orange zest and chopped cilantro in a blender. Slowly add olive oil then sesame oil, blending until creamy. Season with salt and pepper to taste.

INDIAN BROWN RICE PUDDING

Ingredients:

1 Cup of Basmati brown rice (Rinsed and soaked in fresh water for 30 minutes to 1 hour, this reduces the cooking time.)
2 Cups of water
3 Cups of organic coconut mylk
4 Cardomom seeds, crushed
A Pinch of saffron threads or about 1/8 teaspoon
¼ Cup of golden raisins
1-½ Tablespoons of Ghee (or clarified butter, this is optional, but highly recommended.)
2 Tablespoons of unsalted pistachios, peeled and chopped.

Directions:

In a sauce pan, bring the water and the soaked rice to a boil. Reduce the heat to medium low, cover and cook for 20 minutes. Uncover and make sure that all or almost all the water has been absorbed. Add the mylk, stir, cover again and cook on low heat for 15 more minutes. Combine and stir crushed cardamon, saffron and raisins. Cook uncovered for an additional 10 minutes until the rice is tender and most of the mylk has been absorbed. Remove from the heat, add the Ghee and stir gently to combine. Serve in individual bowls and top with the chopped pistachios.

TAHINI FRENCH TOAST GLUTEN-FREE

Ingredients:

6 Slices of gluten free bread
3/4 Cup of almond mylk (or other non-dairy mylk)
3 Large eggs

3 Tablespoons of palm sugar
4 Tablespoons of Ghee
Tahini (sesame paste)
Honey
Ground cinnamon as per taste
Pinch of Himalayan salt

Toast Directions:

In a large shallow bowl, whisk together the almond mylk, eggs and palm sugar until well combined. Dip bread into the mixture, allow to soak for 30 seconds on each side. Remove any excess mixture and set aside on a cooling rack over a baking sheet. Melt 2 tablespoons of Ghee in a non-stick sauté pan over medium low heat. Place 2 slices of bread at a time into the pan and cook until golden brown, approximately 2 to 3 minutes per side. Continue the process with the remaining slices of bread, adding more ghee as necessary. Serve the French toast hot drizzled with tahini and honey, Himalayan salt and a dash of ground cinnamon.

RAW STRAWBERRIES & "CREAM" BANANA FLAX CREPES

Banana Flax Crepes Ingredients:
7 Bananas
½ Cup of ground golden flaxseeds
4 Teaspoons of almond butter
3 Teaspoons of chia seed

Banana Flax Crepes Directions:
Blend bananas into a food processor until creamy. Blend in remaining ingredients. Line dehydrator tray with ParaFlexx Ultra

Sheets. Using a spoon, scoop mixture onto sheet and make round crepes.

Dehydrate for 7-8 hours at 115 degrees, flip the crepes over and dehydrator for an additional hour.

Strawberry Cream Ingredients:

1 Cup of raw cashews that have been soaked overnight
1 Cup of strawberries
½ Cup of spring or filtered water
1 Tablespoon of coconut nectar

Strawberry Cream Directions:

Drain and rinse cashews and place into a food processor. Blend for 20 seconds. Scrape down the sides and blend again. Add water slowly into the food processor. The more water added, the thinner the cream will become. Add coconut nectar and strawberries, blend until creamy.

GRANOLA WITH RAISIN, SEEDS AND FRESH COCONUT MYLK GLUTEN-FREE

Ingredients:

1 Cup of gluten-free raw granola
1-½ cup of coconut or almond mylk
1 Tablespoon of raisins
1 Tablespoon of sunflower seeds

Directions:

Add granola to mylk and top with raisins and seeds.

CAULIFLOWER PANCAKES

Ingredients:

1 Head of cauliflower, chopped

4 Cloves garlic, minced

2 Organic eggs

¼ Cup of spelt flour

1 Teaspoon of almond oil

1 Teaspoon of masala

1 Teaspoon of cumin

Directions:

Boil the cauliflower until soft, drain and place in mixing bowl. Sauté garlic until tender and add cumin, masala and pepper. Pour the garlic mixture over the cauliflower. Add eggs, flour and salt to cauliflower and mix. Heat the almond oil over medium heat in small nonstick pan. Form the cauliflower mixture into pancakes and place one at a time in the pan. Fry for 4 minutes on each side. If you prefer, you can bake at 325 degrees for 30 minutes.

LENTIL SOUP

Ingredients:

2 Teaspoons of Coconut oil

1 Cup of onion, finely chopped

½ Cup of carrot, finely chopped

½ Cup of celery, finely chopped

2 Teaspoons of Himalayan salt

1 Pound of lentils, rinsed and drained

1 Cup of tomatoes, peeled and chopped

2 Quarts of vegetable broth (Non MSG)

½ Teaspoon of coriander powder
Pinch of black pepper (Grains of Paradise)

Directions:

Place the Coconut oil into a large 6 quart Dutch oven and set over medium heat. Once hot, add the onion, carrot, celery and Himalayan salt and cook until the onions are translucent, approximately 6 to 7 minutes. Add and combine the lentils, tomatoes, broth, coriander, cumin and Grains of Paradise. Increase the heat to high and bring to a boil. Reduce the heat to low, cover and cook at a low simmer until the lentils are tender, approximately 35 to 40 minutes. Using a stick blender, puree to preferred consistency. Serve immediately.

ZESTY CORN CAKES

Ingredients:

2 Cups of fresh organic corn kernels or 3 bags organic frozen corn
2 Organic eggs
1 Onion, finely chopped
2 Cloves of garlic, minced
Himalayan salt, pepper and cumin to taste
½ Package raw feta cheese (Add pinch of Himalayan salt if the cheese is not raw.)
2 Tablespoons of Spelt flour

Directions:

Blend all ingredients in a blender and pour the mixture into a baking pan (any size or shape is fine). Bake at 350 degrees for 30 to 45 minutes in the oven or until the top is brown.

TOMATO MISO SOUP

Ingredients:
1 Tomato
4 Tablespoons of Chickpea miso (non-soy miso)
4 Cups of water (115 degrees warmed)
2 Tablespoons of Tocotrienols (A source of Vitamin E powder)
¼ Inch of ginger
¼ Teaspoon of Gram masala
Himalayan salt and pepper to taste

Soup Directions:
Add all the ingredients together and blend until smooth.

VEGAN CARROT CAKE

Cake Ingredients:
2-¼ Cups of spelt flour
3 Teaspoons of cinnamon
½ Teaspoon of nutmeg
1 Teaspoon of Himalayan salt
½ Cup of applesauce
1 Cup of almond mylk
2 Teaspoons of vanilla
1 Cup of maple Syrup
½ Cup of coconut oil
2 Cups of grated carrots (just shy of one pound)

Frosting Ingredients:
½ Cup of raw macadamia nuts (soaked, drained and rinsed)
½ Cup of raw cashews (soaked, drained and rinsed)

¼ Cup of almond mylk

¼ Cup of maple syrup

2 Tablespoons of coconut oil

1 Teaspoon of vanilla

2 Teaspoons of lemon juice

½ Teaspoon of Himalayan salt

Cake Directions:

Preheat oven to 325 and grease a 9x13in baking pan. In a large bowl, whisk together the flour, cinnamon, nutmeg and salt. In a separate bowl, whisk together the applesauce, almond mylk, vanilla, maple and oil. Mix the dry ingredients into the bowl with the wet ingredients. Fold in the carrots and stir until just combined. Bake for 30-40 minutes or until a toothpick comes out clean. Let cake cool completely before frosting.

Frosting Directions:

Combine frosting ingredients in a high speed blender. Start the blender on low and gradually increase the speed, the mixture will be very thick at first. You can add an extra tablespoon of almond mylk if necessary to get your blade moving. Taste and add more maple or lemon to make it sweeter and/or more tangy. Blend until very smooth. Chill for at least 30 minutes before spreading unto the cake. As the frosting cools, it becomes firmer.

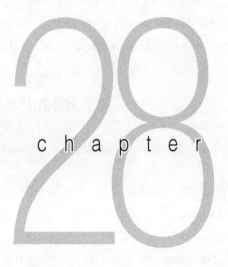

chapter

28

Post – SEXi Juicing _Raw_ Recipes

a s mentioned earlier, you should try to eat 80% raw or uncooked food for as long as possible. There are millions of ways to make raw food easy, fun and tasty. I'm sharing some of my favorite recipes to help you get the most benefits of raw food without compromising delicious flavor.

GINGER-NUT RAW SUSHI

It's helpful to have a bamboo sushi mat for this recipe.

"Rice" Ingredients:
½ Head of cauliflower
½ Carrot
1 Heaping teaspoon of grated ginger
Juice from 1/2 of a lime
1 Heaping teaspoon of almond butter
1 Heaping teaspoon of sunflower butter
1 Heaping teaspoon of tahini

"Rice" Directions:
Place cauliflower and carrot in food processor and pulse until finely chopped into a rice-like texture. Place in a bowl and blend in the rest of ingredients, set aside.

Sushi Ingredients:
Nori or seaweed sheets (1 per person)
Handful of alfalfa sprouts
1 Cucumber julienned
1 Avocado sliced
A few baby spinach leaves
Add in any other vegetables you like

Mix in seasoning such as: Dulce, coriander or fresh herbs.

Sushi Directions:

Before you start to make the sushi, fill a bowl with fresh water and 1/3 cup of rice vinegar. Use this water to wet your hands before making each roll. Put a Nori sheet on a dry surface of cutting board or bamboo sushi mat. First, put a nice layer of alfalfa sprouts, covering nearly half of the Nori sheet. Spread 4 or 5 tablespoons of the "rice" mixture along the edge on top of the sprouts. Make a little indent in the rice and put vegetables on top. Top that with a few pieces of avocado. Finish off with some sunflower or radish sprouts (optional). Roll it up! You can roll the sushi with a bamboo sushi mat or use your fingers. Use your thumbs and finger to roll it up, tightening the roll as you go. Wet the top of the Nori sheet with a little water to seal the sushi. Let the roll sit for 5 minutes before cutting. Using a sharp knife, cut the roll into 5 or 6 equal parts. Use a seesaw motion to make it a perfect, smooth cut. Serve with dipping sauce.

Dipping Sauce Ingredients:

1/8 Cup of lime juice

1/8 Cup of coconut aminos or soy free seasoning sauce

A few drops of stevia, raw honey or coconut nectar

1 Garlic clove, minced.

Dipping Sauce Directions:

Whisk all ingredients together until properly mixed.

KELP NOODLES WITH CREAMY ALMOND SAUCE

Ingredients:

3 Tablespoons of raw almond butter

2 Tablespoons of tahini

2 Garlic cloves

1 Tablespoon of coconut oil

2 Tablespoons of coconut aminos

1-½ Cups of lime juice

1 Teaspoon of Himalayan salt

6 Drops of stevia or small amount of sweetener of choice

1 Teaspoon of coconut vinegar

1 Teaspoon of Brewer's yeast

½ to 1 Tablespoon of grated fresh ginger

Cayenne or chill pepper flakes to taste

½ Teaspoon of cinnamon (or more to taste)

½ Teaspoon of ground coriander

¼ - ½ Cup of water

Chop fresh veggies such as baby bok choy, pea greens, carrots, daikon and bean sprouts.

Directions

Rinse noodles and place in a bowl with water and lemon and let them soak for at least 15 minutes.

Put all ingredients except noodles and chopped veggies in a blender and blend until creamy. Add water until you reach desired creamy consistency. Combine noodles, chopped veggies and sauce in bowl and allow to sit for 10 to 20 minutes before serving.

RED PEPPER-PISTACHIO BISQUE

The nutty, herby Pistou gives this bisque just the right amount of texture. The smooth soup makes a great appetizer or a perfect light lunch.

Bisque Ingredients:
1 Cup of unsweetened almond mylk
1 Cup of filtered water
1 Teaspoon of lemon juice
1 Shallot, peeled and chopped
2 Red Bell Peppers, stemmed, seeded and chopped
1 Serrano pepper (optional), stemmed, seeded and chopped
2 Teaspoon of sweet Hungarian paprika
1 Teaspoon of Himalayan salt to taste
½ Teaspoon of ground cumin
½ Teaspoon of ground cardamom
¼ Cup of raw pistachios, soaked
¼ Cup of raw cashews, soaked
1 Small or ½ large ripe avocado, pitted and peeled

Pistou Ingredients:
½ Cup of packed fresh flat leaf parsley
¼ Cup of dry raw pistachio nuts
1 Tablespoon of Brewer's yeast
1/8 Teaspoon of Himalayan salt to taste
2 Teaspoon of extra virgin olive oil

Directions:
Make Pistou first: Mix parsley, pistachios, Brewer's yeast and salt in a bowl; a mini food processor works best. Pulse until coarsely chopped. Add the olive oil and process until the mixture is finely

chopped and set aside. Bisque directions: Mix all ingredients in a high speed blender adding the avocado last, blend until very smooth. Bisque can be served at room temperature. Chill for a few hours or gently warmed in a dehydrator or oven. Top each serving of soup with ¼ of the reserved pistou that was set aside. Add freshly ground black pepper to taste.

NEW GAZPACHO

Ingredients:

2 or 3 ripe medium tomatoes or 1-½ pints cherry tomatoes
5 or 6 Sun dried tomatoes (soak 1 to 2 hours in advance)
½ Red bell pepper
½ Cup of fresh basil, chopped
1 Cup of cucumber
¼ Cup of chopped red onion
1 Juiced lime
½ Clove of garlic (optional)
A pinch of cayenne pepper (Pepper is spicy hot and is an optional ingredient.)

Directions:

First blend the tomatoes and sun dried tomatoes to an almost liquid consistency. Then add the other ingredients in the order listed, except for the red onion and lightly blend till chunky. Garnish each serving with the chopped red onion.

VEGGIE CRACKERS

These are a super healthy, crunchy and awesome snack!

Ingredients:
1 Cup of carrots
1 Cup of zucchini
1 Small onion
1 Small red pepper
½ Small green pepper
3 Cloves of garlic
1 Cup of soaked almonds (overnight)
1 Cup of ground flaxseeds (golden)
Himalayan salt to taste

Directions:
Finely chop all veggies and almonds in the food processor. Gradually stir in ground flaxseeds until the mixture is smooth. Spread onto dehydrator sheets and place in the dehydrator for 2 hours at a 115 degrees. Cut into rectangular shapes with a pastry wheel and place back in dehydrator for 24 hours.

CHOCOLATE PUDDING

Ingredients:
1 Very ripe avocado
2 or 4 Tablespoons of raw cacao
Sweetener of choice to taste (Coconut nectar, stevia or maple syrup)
Himalayan salt to taste
1 Cup of water or seed mylk as liquid base

Optional additions: Ginger, cayenne, mesquite, maca, soaked raw nuts or shredded coconut.

Directions:

Mix everything in a blender, starting with just a little liquid and sweetener to ensure you don't turn this into a smoothie. I'm crazy with cacao recipes and add all kinds of superfoods, including green powders, maca and others. The amount of cacao depends on how rich tasting you like your chocolate. If you prefer more of a mylk chocolate taste, definitely use a seed mylk base. You can add whole nuts to the blender for a smoother consistency or add whole nuts after for a more crunchy taste.

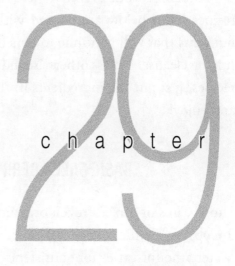

chapter

29

Post – SEXi Juicing Raw
Smoothie Recipes

aw food doesn't mean you have to chew on pieces of kale or celery stalks. An easy and delicious way to incorporate raw foods into your everyday life is to make raw smoothies. The recipes listed below are packed with live enzymes and essential nutrients that will continue to benefit your body after your SEXi Juicing cleanse. Unless otherwise indicated, for all of the following recipes, just put the ingredients in the blender, mix until smooth and enjoy!

BASIC GREEN BERRY SMOOTHIE

1 to 2 Cups of mixed frozen organic berries
2 Cups of organic, mixed baby greens
Water amount varies for consistency preference
Sweetener of choice optional (Coconut nectar, stevia or maple syrup)

POM ALOE MORNING ELIXIR

2 Cups of water
½ Cup of ice cubes
4 Frozen strawberries
1 or 2 Ounces of pomegranate juice
1 Tablespoon of bee pollen
1 Tablespoon of flax or coconut oil
Vanilla stevia to taste
½ of a juiced lemon
1 Heaping teaspoon of tocotrienols (A source of Vitamin E powder)
1 Heaping teaspoon of maca

MORNING POWER SMOOTHIE

1 Banana

½ Cup of frozen organic blueberries

1 Head of butter or red leaf lettuce or a bag of baby or Mesclun lettuce mix

1 Tablespoon of organic raw almond butter

1/3 to ½ cup of unsweetened vanilla almond mylk

½ Cup of additional water, amount varies for consistency preference

½ teaspoon of spirulina

½ Teaspoon of maca powder

1/8 Teaspoon of Himalayan salt

Sweetener of choice optional (Coconut nectar, stevia or maple syrup)

MORNING BANANA START SMOOTHIE

1 Banana

1 or 2 Cups of water or raw seed mylk

1 Teaspoon of maca

½ Teaspoon of mesquite

1 Tablespoon of bee pollen

1 Cup of baby spinach leaves

A dash of Himalayan salt

Sweetener of choice optional (Coconut nectar, stevia or maple syrup)

Also optional: cacao powder, green powder, hemp protein powder, cinnamon, cayenne and/or ice.

CHOCOLATE – BANANA SUPER PUDDING

1 Small or medium frozen banana
2 Teaspoons of raw cacao
½ Teaspoon of maca
½ Teaspoon of spirulina
¼ Cup of water or nut mylk, such as coconut or almond mylk, amount will vary for consistency preference.
Sweetener of choice optional (Coconut nectar, stevia or maple syrup)
1/8 Teaspoon of Himalayan salt (optional)

BEE BERRY MORNING ZINGER

2 Cups of water
Juice of 1 or 2 limes
Juice of 1 orange
1 Heaping teaspoon of bee pollen
1 Inch of ginger root
½ Teaspoon of coconut oil
1 to 2 Teaspoons of goji berries
Sweetener of choice optional (Coconut nectar, stevia or maple syrup)
2 or 3 Cubes of ice

Begin by peeling ginger and putting it in blender to grind. Add the rest of ingredients and enjoy!

BERRY PEARY GREEN SMOOTHIE

1 Apple
1 Pear
½ Cup of blackberries

1 Cup of water
2 Ice cubes
2 Cups of organic spinach
1 Teaspoon of ginger juice or more per your taste
Juice of 1 lime
Also optional: Mint, cilantro, stevia, spirulina and/or cayenne
pepper to taste.

APPLE BERRY GREEN SMOOTHIE

1 Apple
1/3 Cup of frozen organic blackberries
Juice of ½ to 1 whole lime
2 or 3 Kale leaves
A small handful of cilantro
1 Tablespoon of coconut oil
1 Teaspoon of spirulina
Cayenne pepper to taste
Sweetener of choice optional (Coconut nectar, stevia or maple syrup)

VERY BERRY CHOCOLATE SMOOTHIE

5 Ounces of plain organic yogurt
2 Teaspoons of organic raw cacao
1/8 Teaspoons of organic maca
½ Teaspoon of organic vanilla extract
½ Cup of organic frozen blueberries
2 or 4 Ice cubes
1/8 Cup of water, may vary for consistency preference
Pinch of Himalayan salt

COCONUT CITRUS GREEN SMOOTHIE

1 Cup of coconut mylk
½ Large cucumber
1 Lemon juice
2 Clementines
½ Bag of organic herb salad mix
¼ teaspoon of spirulina powder
5 Ice cubes

SLUSHIE SWEET ENERGY SALAD SMOOTHIE

1 Small head of lettuce, chopped
1 Ripe banana
1 Cup of frozen organic blueberries
½ Cup of frozen organic mango
1 Tablespoon of chia seeds
1 to ½ Cup of water

Blend water, lettuce and banana then add frozen fruits and chia seeds. Blend until completely smooth.

VEGETABLE SMOOTHIE

2 Medium tomatoes
½ Medium avocado
6 Romaine lettuce leaves
½ Medium cucumber
2 Tablespoons of lemon juice
½ Cup of water

COOL GREEN SMOOTHIE

2 or 3 Cups of organic spinach
6 Stalks of dandelion greens, tops and bottoms
Juice of 1/2 a lime
1 Inch piece of ginger root
Several ice cubes
1 Cup of water
1 Bunch of mint leaves
Vanilla stevia to taste

GREEN PAPAYA SMOOTHIE

½ Cup of water
2 or 3 cups of fresh or frozen organic papaya
½ Cup of fresh or frozen organic strawberries
2 Bananas
3 Large leaves of Swiss chard without stems.

Blend papaya with water and add other ingredients progressively.
Blend until smooth.

THE GREEN HORNET

6 Organic spinach leaves
2 Cucumbers
½ Bunch of celery
1 Bunch of mint
1 Bunch of flat leaf parsley
2 Green apples
4 Slices of pineapple

Put all the ingredients through a juicer and add whatever supplement you feel you need for the day. Then blend in a blender. Pour the smoothie into a large glass over ice.

RAW SEED MYLK

1 Cup of raw organic seeds, pumpkin, sesame or hemp, pre-soaked overnight
2 Cups of water
Sweetener of choice optional (Coconut nectar, stevia or maple syrup)
Pinch of Himalayan salt.

Place seeds in a large blender filled with water. Blend for one minute. Pour mylk through a strainer bag into a container, pitcher or bowl. When all liquid has gone through the bag, squeeze out any excess fluid and place the pulp in bag aside, to be used at a later time. Add a dash of Himalayan salt. This is your basic nut mylk recipe and will keep 2 or 3 days in the refrigerator. At this point, you have the option of leaving it as is, sweetening and/or flavoring it. To flavor pour back in blender and add sweeteners or flavors of your choice. Suggested flavors: vanilla, cinnamon, cardamom and nutmeg.

SPIRULINA SMOOTHIE

If you are new to spirulina and superfoods in general, I suggest adding them to a smoothie and drinking them every day. Use 1 quart of clean spring water if you can. Add 1 ripe organic banana as a base. Then add 1 teaspoon of spirulina and increase as you get used to the taste. Blend in the following for flavor:

1 Tablespoon of organic raw cacao nibs

1 Handful of raw organic goji berries (Soak in water overnight if you want them to blend more smoothly.)

½ to 1 Tablespoon of organic raw maca powder

½ to 1 Tablespoon of lucuma powder

1 Tablespoon of bee pollen, whole granules

½ to 1 Teaspoon of organic ginger root powder

VANILLA NUT SMOOTHIE

1 Cup of young coconut water

½ Cup of packed young coconut pulp

1/3 Cup of macadamia nuts

½ to ¾ Cup of ice

¼ Teaspoon of pure vanilla extract

¼ Teaspoon of Lucuma powder (Maple tasting, low glycemic sweetener from a Peruvian Lucuma fruit.)

1/8 Teaspoon of mesquite powder

Sweetener of choice optional (Coconut nectar, stevia or maple syrup)

Vanilla stevia to taste

chapter

Post – SEXi Juicing *Juice* Recipes

All of the following juice recipes should be made with organic fresh or frozen fruits and vegetables when possible.

JOLLY GINGER

1 Apple
2 Carrots
1 Celery stalk
1 Inch of ginger root

VEG-TANG TONIC

4 Carrots
2 Celery stalks
1 Handful of parsley
4 Spinach leaves

CBS TONIC

3 Carrots
½ of a Beet
3 Spinach leaves

CITRUS DELIGHT

1 Orange
¼ of a Lemon
¼ of a Grapefruit, peeled

TIP TOP TONIC

1 Apple
4 Carrots

CARROT CLEANSER

3 Carrots
½ of a Beet
½ of a Cucumber

GINGER ZINGER

3 Carrots
1 Stalk of celery
1 Handful of parsley
1 Clove of garlic
1 Apple
4 Carrots
1 Inch of ginger root

FAB FRUIT COCKTAIL

2 Apples
1 Cup of cranberries
1 Bunch of grapes

TOMATO SURPRISE

1 Tomato
2 Large carrots

TROPICAL ENVY

½ of a Beet
2 Carrots
1 Stalk celery
½ of a Cucumber
1 Inch of ginger root
1 Handful of parsley
2 Slices of pineapple

RED EYE

3 Carrots
½ of a Beet
1 Clove of garlic
1 Inch of ginger root
2 Scallions

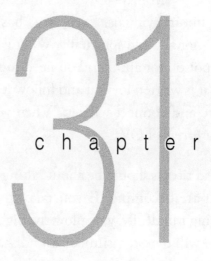

chapter

Final Thoughts On Food

my teacher/Guru, Homeopathic, Spiritual Writer, Medical Doctor Gabriel Cousens, says that food is "a love more from G-D." We all have different notes, because we are bio-individuals. Each of us has a unique makeup physically, emotionally and spiritually. What is nourishing for one person can be poison for another. You need to recognize your own love note, what is written for you and follow it. You need to respect your love note and connect with it. When you connect to your love note, you *become* LOVE.

Food rituals should be about taking time to connect with whoever you are becoming. If you take time for yourself, you will start eating mindfully, you allow the digestive process to start correctly. You will digest, assimilate and discard your food the right way. If on the other hand, you eat on the run, you can produce a fight-or-flight reaction. Your body's energies are not in the digestive tract but in your brain or feet. You will not be able to digest your food properly. You will develop constipation, gas, bloating and/or acid reflux because you are on your cell phone and computer, constantly receiving negative information and energy from electronic gadgets that surround you most of the day.

So, for your next meal, prepare a nice table, light a candle if you wish, write your love from G-D and sit down to connect with and respect the food you have prepared. Say a blessing or a mantra, raise the vibration of the food to your body and eat slowly. Take time to chew. Put your fork down between bites. When you chew food well, you will recognize your body's signals that you are getting full and you will stop. You will eat less as a result. Remember that quality food will be satisfying for your body, resulting in consuming smaller quantities. Always ask yourself, "Is this quality food or quantity food?" Stop supersizing your food.

You are overwhelming your body and enlarging your organs, making you age faster. You are the best, so have the best, and don't be satisfied with less than that.

If you're eating with others, take time to really connect with them, heart-to-heart.

Eat breakfast like a king or a queen. Lunch like a prince or a princess and dinner like a college student with a maxed out credit card.

The yogis say that your stomach should be divided into three parts. The first part should be filled with lukewarm water sipped through the meal, the second part with food and the third part should remain empty. You should always ask yourself while you eat, "Am I satisfied, hungry or full?" You should be able to stop anywhere between satisfied and full. Never reach the point of feeling stuffed. Stuffed people are the ones who get sick and age prematurely.

When you eat slowly, calmly savor every bite and appreciate the food, you will be able to shift your life from focusing on your obsession to finding your passions. It will happen organically. As a result, you will find your higher purpose. For me, higher purpose is being in service to other people. By giving, you reach beyond yourself, beyond your personal needs and focus on the community and world around you. By doing so, you actually receive so much in return.

Hindu Goddess Bhavani said; "We truly experience love when we can fully, openly, unconditionally and without limitation letting ourselves be loving." We have it all within us and the greatest gift anyone can give us is welcoming and receiving our love. It's an almost miraculous transformation, the magic that happens when you turn a situation around and concentrate on loving - just love on loving - not on needing or wanting or longing to be loved. LOVE IS THE LOVING. I wish with all my heart that if you haven't yet discovered this feeling, you will soon. If you have relished in this extraordinary feeling of bliss, then you already know how boundless love is.

I wish you all peace, happiness, health and an open, loving heart!

Amen,
Dr. Etti

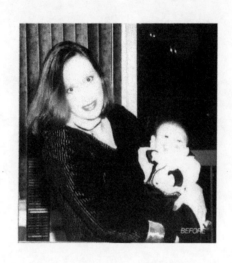

appendix a

Pre-Juicing Assessment

Before you start the SEXi Juicing journey, I want you to assess where you are right now. We will revisit these same questions when you complete the program. You will find the Post Juicing Assessment in Appendix B.

What is your current weight?

How do you feel in the following ways most of the time? Rate the following from 1 to 10 (1= very low and 10= very high).

Energy level:

Stress level:

Overall health and well-being level:

Self confidence level:

Satisfaction with health:

Satisfaction with work:

Satisfaction with relationships:

Satisfaction with life:

List four things you would like to accomplish as a result of the SEXi Juicing program:

How would a successful outcome make you feel?

What are some potential obstacles?

How do you plan to overcome these obstacles?

Who can you call for support during the seven day SEXI Juicing program?

Is there someone in your life that you can count on to hold you accountable to REACH your goals? Let them know that you are starting your SEXi Juicing adventure. Ask them to support you and your journey by checking in with you daily, encouraging when you get weak or about to falter and celebrating with you when you reach your goal. Write the name of your SEXi Juicing buddy or buddies below:

Name: Relationship:

Name: Relationship:

Name: Relationship:

Remember, the person accountable at all times is *you*.

Support yourself through affirmations, meditation and visualization.

Post - Juicing Assessment

Congratulations for completing the seven day SEXi Juicing journey! Take time to fill in this Post-Juicing Assessment and compare it to your Pre-Juicing Assessment from Appendix A. By comparing the Pre-Juicing and Post-Juicing Assessments you will clearly see your successes and be motivated to power through your post cleanse phase. Achieving balance and health is a lifelong journey.

What is your current weight?

How do you feel most of the time? Rate the following from 1 to 10 (1 = very low and 10 = very high):

- Energy level:
- Stress level:
- Overall health and well-being level:
- Self-confidence level:
- Satisfaction with health:
- Satisfaction with work:
- Satisfaction with relationships:
- Satisfaction with life:

List four things you accomplished as a result of the SEXi Juicing program.

What was the most challenging part of the SEXi Juicing program?

What was the most enjoyable part of the SEXi Juicing program?

What do you want to maintain from the SEXi Juicing program?

What old habits do you want to release?

What food or drink do you want to eliminate from your diet?

What food or drink do you want to add to your diet?

What self-care activities do you want to add to your daily routine?

appendix c

PUMKIN SEEDS

Pumpkin seeds are among the few foods that contain zinc, which are vital for testosterone production in men. Similarly, women who are zinc deficient can completely lose their sex drive. These yummy seeds are also a rich source of omega-3 fatty-acids, which are vital to overall sexual well-being, reduce inflammation and may help lower the risk of chronic diseases, i.e. heart, cancer and arthritis.

GOJI BERRIES

In Asia, goji berries are considered a strong sexual food. They increase testosterone levels, which stimulates libido in men and women. Furthermore, they improve stamina, mood and well-being, all of which are vital for an optimum sex life.

MACA

One of the new superfoods, this root vegetable and medicinal herb is valued because it can improve sexual performance and alleviate impotence. It increases sperm count and testosterone levels in men and increases sexual desire, particularly in women.

BANANAS

These easy to find fruits boosts male libido, thanks to an enzyme called bromelain, which is important to sexual health. They are also a good source of B vitamins, which increase the body's energy level and sex hormones.

CELERY

This sexual stimulator boosts the level of a powerful steroid hormone known as androsterone, an odorless aphrodisiac in male perspiration, made in the liver from the metabolism of testosterone.

AVOCADOS
Avocados help increase male and female libidos. They contain very high levels of folic acid and promote sexual energy. They are also loaded with vitamin B6, a potent hormone regulator.

BEE POLLEN
Bee pollen can help boost sperm count, which is not surprising since it is made from millions of particles of a semen-like substance and its role in nature is to fertilize.

Foods to Enhance Your SEXi Self

ASPARAGUS
Asparagus boasts an abundance of Vitamin E, a vital nutrient for good sex and is loaded with folate (folic acid) and potassium. In addition, its stalks contain large amounts of antioxidants.

CHILES
Capsaicin, is the substance that gives chilies their heat, releases endorphins and other "feel good" hormones necessary for a spicy sex life.

BASIL
Basil increases circulation, stimulates sex drive and boosts fertility. This tasty herb cultivates a sense of well-being, which allows one to experience sexual bliss.

FIGS
Figs are very rich in amino acids which are critical to increasing libido and boosting sexual stamina.

GARLIC
Finely chopped garlic contains high levels of allicin which can improve blood flow to the sexual organs.

RAW CACAO
Cacao (ka-cow) is the raw, unprocessed from of chocolate. The untreated seeds, referred to as cacao beans, are a superfood offering a wealth of antioxidants, essential vitamins and minerals.

Cacao beans grow on small trees called Theobroma cacao, which literally translates to, "cacao, the food of the gods." These trees are native to Mexico, Central and South America. Each cacao pod that emerges from the tree typically houses between 40 to 60 cacao seeds. After careful harvesting, the pods are opened, the seeds are removed to undergo a natural fermentation and drying process. After the drying process is completed in 1-2 weeks, you are left with raw cacao beans.

To make the chocolate that we all know and love, these raw cacao beans are roasted to form cocoa, which is then combined with sugar and fats until the beans are unrecognizable. The high heat in the roasting process reduces the levels of antioxidants in the cacao, minimizing the powerful health benefits found in the unprocessed, raw cacao.

To receive the greatest benefits from cacao, look for raw, non-roasted cacao beans

Foods to Enhance Your SEXi Self

RAW CACAO HEALTH BENEFITS

Raw cacao contains many important vitamins and minerals, including:

- Magnesium, calcium, sulfur, zinc, iron, copper, potassium and manganese
- Polyphenols called flavonoids, with antioxidant properties
- Vitamins B1, B2, B3, B5, B9 and E
- Essential heart healthy fat, oleic acid, a monounsaturated fat
- Protein
- Fiber

These nutrients found in raw cacao have been linked to a number of health benefits:

Lowers Blood Pressure and Improves Circulation

Cacao helps thin the blood, thus slowing coagulation. In a study of healthy individuals who consumed a strong cacao beverage, platelet aggregation was reduced and fewer micro-particles than normally formed. Additionally, the test subjects' blood took longer to form a clot than blood taken from those individuals who had not consumed the cocoa beverage.

Promotes Cardiovascular Function and Health

Polyphenols are reportedly cardio-protective in two ways. First, they help reduce oxidation of low density lipoproteins (LDL), the so called "bad cholesterol" which are considered a major threat to heart health, most notably from heart attacks and strokes. Polyphenols also inhibit blood platelets from clumping together. This clumping process, called aggregation, can lead to atherosclerosis, which is also known as hardening of the arteries. By inhibiting aggregation, polyphenols reduce the risk of atherosclerosis. Since atherosclerosis is a major killer of American adults, the protection provided by the polyphenols in cacao is of real value.

Neutralizes Free Radicals

High levels of antioxidants protect the body from a buildup of free radicals from sun exposure, pollution, cigarette smoke and et cetera, which may damage healthy body tissue, giving rise to cancer and cardiovascular diseases.

Improves Digestion

A sufficient amount of fiber delivered with each serving of cacao supports digestion while cacao stimulates the body's production of digestive enzymes.

Enhances Physical, Sexual and Mental Well-Being

The multitude of compounds in cocoa, phenethylamine (or PEA) may be one of the most valuable. Phenethylamine stimulates the nervous system and triggers the release of pleasurable opium like compounds known as endorphins. It also kick starts the activity of dopamine, a neurochemical directly associated with sexual arousal and pleasure. In addition, phenethylamine increases in the brain when we fall in love and during orgasms.

Additionally, Cacao promotes a sense of well-being by increasing serotonin, the so called feel-good chemical in the brain. For this reason, cacao and chocolate can provide a highly desirable mood boost to women during PMS and menstruation, when serotonin levels are often low. In fact, women are consistently more sensitive to chocolate than men and typically experience stronger chocolate cravings than men.

a p p e n d i x   d

Bonus Receipes

DR ETTI'S SEXi LOVE CHOCOPOTION

Ingredients:

1 Teaspoon of raw cacao powder

½ Teaspoon of cacao nibs

1 Cup of filtered water, (not tap water)

2 Cup of non-dairy mylk, but not soy mylk

Sweeten to taste using xylitol, honey, stevia or SweetE

1 Pinch of Himalayan salt

Directions:

Place all ingredients in a blender and mix for 30 seconds. You can make this drink with ice or as hot coco. It is best to stop drinking Dr Etti's Love Chocopotion four hours before bedtime.

DR. ETTI'S SEXi LEMONADE OR LIMONADE

Ingredients:

2 Lemons or limes, peeled without ring

2 Cups of mineral water

Sweeten to taste using xylitol, honey, stevia or SweetE

3 Fresh mint leaves (optional)

4 Large Ice cubes

Directions:

Blend all ingredients on high for 30 seconds.

a p p e n d i x   e

Song Lyrics

"MICHAEL, ROW THE BOAT ASHORE"
By William Francis Allen, Charles Pickard
Ware and Lucy McKim Garrison

Michael, row the boat ashore, hallelujah.
Michael, row the boat ashore, hallelujah.

My brothers and sisters are all aboard, hallelujah.
My brothers and sisters are all aboard, hallelujah.
Michael, row the boat ashore, hallelujah.
Michael, row the boat ashore, hallelujah.

The river is deep and the river is wide, hallelujah.
Mylk and honey on the other side, hallelujah.
Michael, row the boat ashore, hallelujah.
Michael, row the boat ashore, hallelujah.

Jordan's river is chilly and cold, hallelujah.
Chills the body but not the soul, hallelujah.
Michael, row the boat ashore, hallelujah.
Michael, row the boat ashore, hallelujah.
Michael, row the boat ashore, hallelujah.

My brothers and sisters are all abroad, hallelujah.
My brothers and sisters are all aboard, hallelujah
Michael, row the boat ashore, hallelujah.
Michael, row the boat ashore, hallelujah.

The river is deep and the river is wide, hallelujah.
Mylk and honey on the other side, hallelujah.
Michael, row the boat ashore, hallelujah.
Michael, row the boat ashore, hallelujah.

Jordan's river is chilly and cold, hallelujah.
Chills the body but not the soul, hallelujah.
Michael, row the boat ashore, hallelujah.
Michael, row the boat ashore, hallelujah.

Song Lyrics

"ROW, ROW, ROW YOUR BOAT"
By: Eliphalet Oram Lyte

Row, row, row your boat,
Gently down the stream.
Merrily, merrily, merrily, merrily,
Life is but a dream.

"SEXUAL HEALING"
By: David Ritz, Odell Brown and Marvin Gaye

Whenever blue teardrops are fallin',
And my emotional stability is leaving me,
There is something I can do,
I can get on the telephone and call you up baby.

appendix f

Frequently Asked Questions

Do I need to prepare for the SEXi Juicing cleanse?

Yes, take time over the next 48 hours to simplify your diet and plan for your SEXi Juicing cleanse. If you have just purchased this book, you have a couple of days until you start your SEXi Juicing cleanse.

Focus on consuming raw, organic fruits and veggies during this time to increase the benefits and effectiveness of your SEXi Juicing cleanse. Avoid dairy, meat and flour products, such as; pancakes, bread, muffins, cookies and tortillas. Instead, go for cooked whole grains and legumes (for detailed information refer to Chapter 17).

Will I gain all my weight back after doing the SEXi Juicing cleanse?

The answer to this question is simple, it's up to you. If you follow thoroughly SEXi Juicing Part VI: AFTER THE CLEANSE, and continue introducing fresh, organic foods and thoughts to your body, mind and spirit, you will not gain the weight back, but rather continue losing the weight of waste. Cleansing changes things on the inside where real change must begin. You have exercised authority over food, regained self-confidence and accomplished something never thought possible. Here you are, standing before the mirror feeling good about yourself for the first time in years. It's potent stuff, just the boost necessary to start living a fresh, energized determined life. SEXi Juicing is about healthy beginnings, not a quick fix.

People tend to think only of animal products as providing protein but many plant based food, beet greens, broccoli and kale, just to name a few, contain a surprisingly high amount of protein. Your body has sufficient protein reserves for at least a 30 day water fast if not longer. Remember, organic fruit and vegetable juice cleansing is a natural process.

Should I continue with my medication?

It is wise to consult your doctor regarding the possible effect of doing a juice cleanse combined with your medication. Many people can do a successful cleanse while on medication. I, Dr. Etti, am NOT a Medical Doctor and do not claim to treat any illnesses.

The instructions, information and advice contained in this book are for educational purposes only. The content of this book cannot be relied upon as a preventative cure or treatment for any disease or medical condition. It is recommended that you consult with a licensed medical doctor or physician before acting upon any recommendation that is made in this book. Use of this material and the information contained in this book is at your own risk. Dr. Etti does not represent or endorse the accuracy, correctness or reliability of any opinions, statements or information presented in this material.

Dr. Etti is not responsible for any adverse effects or consequences of any kind resulting from the use or misuse of any suggestions, advice, information or instructions described within this book. reader of these materials assumes all risks from the use, non-use or misuse of this information.

This book contains general information about alternative treatments. The information is not advice and should not be treated as such.

The information in this book is provided "as is" without any representations or warranties, expressed or implied. Dr. Etti makes no representations or warranties in relations to the information in this book.

Without prejudice to the generality of the foregoing paragraph, Dr. Etti does not warrant that the information in this book is complete, true, accurate, up-to-date or non-misleading.

Professional assistance
You must not rely on the information in this book as an alternative to medical advice from your doctor or other professional healthcare providers.

If you have any specific questions about any medical matter, you should consult your doctor or other professional healthcare provider.

If you think you might be suffering from any medical condition, you should seek immediate medical attention.

You should never delay seeking medical advice, disregard medical advice or discontinue medical treatment because of information in this book.

How much weight will I lose?
Depends on how toxic and overweight you are, weight loss can initially be as high as three to four pounds per day because much of it is water. As the fast continues, the average loss will be approximately one pound per day because the slower your metabolism, the slower your weight loss.

Remember, your goal should be to lose the weight of waste – Toxic weight.

Will I get too thin?
If you are thin to start with, cleansing may allow you to gain additional weight afterwards. Metabolism is normalized due to the

cleansing process. It is very important not to try to gain weight too quickly. The body can rebuild only at a set rate. Overeating will burden the body and undermine the rebuilding process.

Since I have finished fasting, why am I more sensitive to unhealthy food?

After finishing a SEXi Juicing program, your body is clean and has far less tolerance to the poisonous foods that you were eating prior to the cleansing. Feeling sick when eating junk food is a sign that our body is functioning normally. SEXi Juicing restores the body's ability to violently react to harmful and unhealthy food.

Are there any conditions that restrict juice cleansing?

Yes. The need for expert assistance is especially true when dealing with hypoglycemia (low blood sugar level), diabetes, kidney disease, drug addiction or undergoing chemotherapy.

Can pregnant women cleanse?

It is not recommended for pregnant women or nursing mothers to do a juice cleanse.

Should I abstain from sexual relations during the SEXi Juicing cleanse?

Sexual relations could be distracting. During the first three days, your body is going through a deep, cellular cleans and better utilizes its energy when you're abstain from intercourse.

Can I have more than four servings of juice?

Yes you can. You "eat" your "liquid food" every 3 hours to maintain normal blood sugar levels. If you want one or more servings, please do so. And make sure to hydrate with good quality water, herbal teas or "decorated water" by adding lemon, stevia, salt, turmeric or cayenne pepper. You can also make one more serving of DR.

ETTI'S SEXi LOVE CHOCOPOTION drink (See the recipe in Appendix D).

What possible side effects of cleaning I might experience?

Depends how toxic you are. For the first two or three days, detoxification is at its most drastic and noticeable, as the body adjusts to the new regime. Even though SEXi Juicing is a short term gentle cleanse, you might experience some side effects and withdrawals like: feeling under the weather, minor skin blemishes, headaches, fatigue and/or temporary insomnia. The more pleasant results of SEXi Juicing are soon to follow and usually include healthier looking skin, clear eyes, better awareness of the effects of certain foods on the body, weight loss, clarity of mind, improved digestion, an overall sense of well-being and positive mood.

Remember to listen to your body! Consult a doctor if any of these symptoms begin to interfere with your everyday life or gets worse.

BIBLIOGRAPHY

Aaker, Jennifer, Roy Baumeister, Kathleen Vohs, and Emily Garbinsky. "Stanford Research: The Meaningful Life Is a Road worth Traveling." Stanford University. 1 Jan. 2014. Web. 20 Mar. 2015.

Airola, Paavo O. How to Keep Slim, Healthy and Young with Juice Fasting. Phoenix: Health Plus, 1971. Print.

"Albert Einstein Quotes." *Http://www.brainyquote.com/quotes/authors/a/albert_einstein.html.* Web. 24 Mar. 2015.

Anderson, Richard. *Cleanse & Purify Thyself.* Rev. ed. Medford, Or.: Christobe Pub., 2007. Print.

Annie Hall. Dir. Charles H. Joffe. By Woody Allen and Diane Keaton. MGM Home Entertainment, 2000. DVD.

Barks, Coleman. *The Essential Rumi "Fasting".* San Francisco, CA: Harper, 1995. Print.

Bragg, Paul Chappuis, and Patricia Bragg. *The Miracle of Fasting Proven through History for Physical, Mental and Spiritual Rejuvenation.* 50th ed. Santa Barbara, Calif.: Health Science, 2004. Print.

Cousens, Gabriel. *Conscious Eating.* 2nd ed. Berkeley, Calif.: North Atlantic, 2000. Print.

Dyer, Wayne W. *The Power of Intention: Learning to Co-create Your World Your Way.* Carlsbad, Calif.: Hay House, 2004. Print.

"Elisabeth Kübler-Ross Foundation -." Elisabeth Kübler-Ross Foundation. N.p., n.d. Web. 18 Mar. 2015.u

Gaye, Marvin. *Sexual Healing.* Delta Music, 1996. CD.

Genesis 8 1:31." *The Holy Bible, Containing the Old Testament and the New.* Oxford: U of Oxford: Printed by John Baskett, 1719. Print.Group, Edward F. *Health Begins in the Colon.* Houston, TX: Global Healing Center, 2007. Print.

Hawkins, Dr. David R. *Power vs. Force: The Hidden Determinants of Human Behavior.* Rev. ed. Carlsbad, Calif.: Hay House, 2002. Print.

Hawkins, Dr. David R. *Healing and Recovery.* W. Sedona, AZ: Veritas Pub., 2009. Print

Hofmekler, Ori. "Can You Stop Physical Aging?" Defense Nutrition. 28 Oct. 2011. Web. 20 Mar. 2015.

Katz, Dr. David. "How Modifying What We Do With Our Feet, Forks and Fingers Can Change Our Fate | Big Think." Big Think. N.p., 21 July 2009. Web. 20 Mar. 2015.

Kacera, Walter. *Ayurvedic Tongue Diagnosis.* Twin Lakes, Wis.: Lotus, 2006. Print.

Lama, Dalai The. *"Teaching and Long Life Offering at Palpung Sherabling Monastery." His Holiness the 14ᵗʰ Dalai Lama. N.p., n.d. Web. 18 Mar. 2015.*

Longo, Valter D. "Faculty Profile." USC Davis School of Gerontology. N.p., n.d. Web. 18 Mar. 2015.

Mercola, Dr. Joseph. "Is It Healthy to Skip Breakfast? | Intermittent Fasting." Mercola.com. 4 May 2011. Web. 20 Mar. 2015.

Michael, Row the Boat Ashore. EMI Records, 1992. CD

Mitchell, Gregory. "Carl Jung and Jungian Analytical Psychology." *Carl Jung and Jungian Analytical Psychology*. N.p., n.d. Web. 27 May 2015.

Nepo, Mark. "Mark Nepo - Spiritual Writer, Poet, Philosopher, Healing Arts Teacher, Cancer Survivor." *Mark Nepo - Spiritual Writer, Poet, Philosopher, Healing Arts Teacher, Cancer Survivor*. Web. 22 Mar. 2015.

Nichopoulos, George, and Rose Clayton Phillips. *The King and Dr. Nick: What Really Happened to Elvis and Me*. Nashville: Thomas Nelson, 2009. Print.

"Nithyananda.org." Nithyananda.org. N.p., n.d. Web. 18 Mar. 2015.

"Quote By Abraham Lincoln." *Quotery*. 10 Apr. 2013. Web. 24 Mar. 2015.

Rosenthal, Joshua. "Search." Institute for Integrative Nutrition. 26 Mar. 2008. Web. 20 Mar. 2015.

Sexy [Def. 1]. (n.d.). Merriam-Webster Online. In Merriam-Webster. Retrieved March 18, 2015, from http://www.merriam-webster.com/dictionary/sexy.

Super Size Me. Dir. Morgan Spurlock. 2004. DVD.

Suszynsk, Marie, and Niya Jones, MD, MPH. "Live Longer With Enough Sleep." *EverydayHealth.com*. N.p., n.d. Web. 26 May 2015.

The Matrix. Prod. Andy Wachowski and Lana Wachowski. Dir. Andy Wachowski and Lana Wachowski. By Andy Wachowski and Lana Wachowski. 1999.

"The 50 Best Quotes About Health & Nutrition." Dr. Groups Natural Health Organic Living Blog. N.p., 14 July 2011. Web. 20 Mar. 2015.

The Secret. TS Production, LLC, 2006. DVD.

"Tony Robbins - Official Website of Tony Robbins." Tony Robbins. N.p., n.d. Web. 18 Mar. 2015.

Trapani, Iza, and Steve Blane. Row, Row, Row Your Boat. Scholastic, 2000. CD.

Walia, Arjun. "Fascinating Evidence Shows Why Water Fasting Could Be One Of The Healthiest Things You Can Do." *The Mind Unleashed*. N.p., 14 Apr. 2015. Web. 26 May 2015.

When Harry Met Sally--. Dir. Rob Reiner. 1989

www.ncbi.nlm.nih.gov. Web. 24 Mar. 2015.

Z'ak Z'enu: "Ehyeh Asher Ehyeh" Tel Hai: Omanut Tel Hai, 1999. Print.

Ziglar, Zig. Great Quotes from Zig Ziglar. Franklin Lakes, NJ: Career, 1997. Print.

CPSIA information can be obtained
at www.ICGtesting.com
Printed in the USA
LVHW110939280419
615845LV00001B/237/P